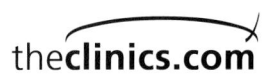

ORTHOPEDIC CLINICS OF NORTH AMERICA

The Pediatric Hip

GUEST EDITOR
James T. Guille, MD

April 2006 • Volume 37 • Number 2

SAUNDERS

An Imprint of Elsevier, Inc.
PHILADELPHIA LONDON TORONTO MONTREAL SYDNEY TOKYO

W.B. SAUNDERS COMPANY
A Division of Elsevier Inc.

Elsevier Inc., 1600 John F. Kennedy Blvd., Suite 1800, Philadelphia, PA 19103-2899.

http://www.orthopedic.theclinics.com

ORTHOPEDIC CLINICS OF NORTH AMERICA
April 2006
Editor: Debora Dellapena

Volume 37, Number 2
ISSN 0030-5898
ISBN 1-4160-3538-9

Copyright © 2006 by Elsevier Inc. All rights reserved. No part of this publication may be reproduced or transmitted in any form or by any means, electronic or mechanical, including photocopy, recording, or any information retrieval system, without written permission from the Publisher.

Single photocopies of single articles may be made for personal use as allowed by national copyright laws. Permission of the Publisher and payment of a fee is required for all other photocopying, including multiple or systematic copying, copying for advertising or promotional purposes, resale, and all forms of document delivery. Special rates are available for educational institutions that wish to make photocopies for non-profit educational classroom use. Permissions may be sought directly from Elsevier's Rights Department in Philadelphia, PA, USA: phone (+1) 215 239 3804, fax (+1) 215 239 3805, e-mail healthpermissions@elsevier.com. Requests may also be completed on-line via the Elsevier homepage (http://www.elsevier.com/locate/permissions). In the USA, users may clear permissions and make payments through the Copyright Clearance Center, Inc., 222 Rosewood Drive, Danvers, MA 01923, USA; phone: (978) 750-8400, fax: (978) 750-4744, and in the UK through the Copyright Licensing Agency Rapid Clearance Service (CLARCS), 90 Tottenham Court Road, London W1P 0LP, UK; phone (+44) 171 436 5931; fax: (+44) 171 436 3986. Other countries may have a local reprographic rights agency for payments.

The ideas and opinions expressed in *Orthopedic Clinics of North America* do not necessarily reflect those of the Publisher. The Publisher does not assume any responsibility for any injury and/or damage to persons or property arising out of or related to any use of the material contained in this periodical. The reader is advised to check the appropriate medical literature and the product information currently provided by the manufacturer of each drug to be administered to verify the dosage, the method and duration of administration, or contraindications. It is the responsibility of the treating physician or other health care professional, relying on independent experience and knowledge of the patient, to determine drug dosages and the best treatment for the patient. Mention of any product in this issue should not be construed as endorsement by the contributors, editors, or the Publisher of the product or manufacturers' claims.

Orthopedic Clinics of North America (ISSN 0030-5898) is published quarterly (For Post Office use only: Volume 37 issue 2 of 4) by W.B. Saunders, 360 Park Avenue South, New York, NY 10010-1710. Months of publication are January, April, July, and October. Business and Editorial Offices: 1600 John F. Kennedy Blvd., Suite 1800, Philadelphia, PA 19103-2899. Accounting and circulation offices: 6277 Sea Harbor Drive, Orlando, FL 33887-4800. Periodicals postage paid at New York, NY and additional mailing offices. Subscription prices are $190.00 per year for (US individuals), $315.00 per year for (US institutions), $225.00 per year (Canadian individuals), $370.00 per year (Canadian institutions), $260.00 per year (international individuals), $370.00 per year (international institutions), $95.00 per year (US students), $130.00 per year (Canadian and international students). Foreign air speed delivery is included in all *Clinics* subscription prices. All prices are subject to change without notice. **POSTMASTER:** Send address changes to *Orthopedic Clinics of North America*, Elsevier Periodicals Customer Service, 6277 Sea Harbor Drive, Orlando, FL 32887-4800. **Customer Service: 1-800-654-2452 (US). From outside of the US, call 1-407-345-4000. E-mail: hhspcs@harcourt.com.**

Reprints. For copies of 100 or more, of articles in this publication, please contact the Commercial Reprints Department, Elsevier Inc., 360 Park Avenue South, New York, New York 10010-1710. Tel. (212) 633-3813 Fax: (212) 462-1935 e-mail: reprints@elsevier.com

Orthopedic Clinics of North America is covered in *Index Medicus, Cinahl, Excerpta Medica, and Cumulative Index to Nursing and Allied Health Literature.*

Printed in the United States of America.

GUEST EDITOR

JAMES T. GUILLE, MD, Orthopaedic Surgeon, Pediatric Orthopaedics and Spinal Deformity, Shriners Hospital for Children, Philadelphia, Pennsylvania

CONTRIBUTORS

JAMES H. BEATY, MD, Professor, Department of Orthopaedic Surgery, University of Tennessee; Chief of Staff, Campbell Clinic, Memphis, Tennessee

RANDAL R. BETZ, MD, Chief of Staff, Shriners Hospital for Children; Professor, Department of Orthopaedic Surgery, Temple University, Philadelphia, Pennsylvania

J. RICHARD BOWEN, MD, Nemours Professor of Orthopaedics, Education, and Research; Attending Surgeon, Alfred I. duPont Hospital for Children, Wilmington, Delaware

GILBERT CHAN, MD, Research Fellow, Department of Orthopaedics, Alfred I. duPont Hospital for Children, Wilmington, Delaware

TAE-JOON CHO, MD, Associate Professor, Department of Orthopedic Surgery, Seoul National University Hospital, Seoul, Korea

IN HO CHOI, MD, Professor, Department of Orthopedic Surgery, Seoul National University Hospital, Seoul, Korea

CHIN YOUB CHUNG, MD, Professor, Department of Orthopedic Surgery, Seoul National University Hospital, Seoul, Korea

MARCIN DOMZALSKI, MD, Assistant, Clinic of Orthopaedics and Pediatric Orthopaedics, Medical University of Lodz, Lodz, Poland

CRAIG P. EBERSON, MD, Assistant Professor, Brown Medical School, Department of Orthopaedics, Hasbro Children's Hospital, Providence, Rhode Island

DANIEL C. FIGUEIREDO, MD, Orthopedic Surgeon, Clinical Fellow of Orthopedics, Hospital Pequeno Príncipe, Curitiba, Brazil

JOHN M. FLYNN, MD, Associate Professor of Orthopaedic Surgery, University of Pennsylvania School of Medicine; Division of Orthopaedic Surgery, Children's Hospital of Philadelphia, Philadelphia, Pennsylvania

EDILSON FORLIN, MD, MSc, PhD, Pediatric Orthopedic Surgeon, Hospital Pequeno Principe and Hospital das Clinicas da UFPR, Curitiba, Brazil; President, Brazilian Pediatric Orthopedic Society, Sao Paulo, Brazil

STEVEN L. FRICK, MD, Director, Pediatric Orthopaedics and Residency Program, Carolinas Medical Center, Charlotte, North Carolina

H. THEODORE HARCKE, MD, Professor, Departments of Radiology and Pediatrics, Jefferson Medical College, Philadelphia, Pennsylvania; Alfred I. duPont Hospital for Children, Wilmington, Delaware

MININDER S. KOCHER, MD, MPH, Associate Director, Division of Sports Medicine, Department of Orthopaedic Surgery, Children's Hospital; Assistant Professor of Orthopaedic Surgery, Harvard Medical School, Harvard School of Public Health, Boston, Massachusetts

S. JAY KUMAR, MD, Clinical Professor of Orthopaedics, Thomas Jefferson University, Philadelphia, Pennsylvania; Attending Surgeon, Department of Orthopaedics, Alfred I. duPont Hospital for Children, Wilmington, Delaware

BEN LEE, BA, Department of Orthopaedic Surgery, Children's Hospital; Harvard Medical School, Boston, Massachusetts

MARK C. LEE, MD, Resident, Brown Medical School, Department of Orthopaedics, Rhode Island Hospital, Providence, Rhode Island

RANDALL T. LODER, MD, Garceau Professor of Pediatric Orthopaedic Surgery, Indiana University School of Medicine; Director, Pediatric Orthopaedics, James Whitcomb Riley Children's Hospital, Indianapolis, Indiana

JAMES J. McCARTHY, MD, Assistant Chief of Staff, Shriners Hospital for Children; Associate Professor, Department of Orthopaedic Surgery, Temple University, Philadelphia, Pennsylvania

LUIZ A. MUNHOZ da CUNHA, MD, MSc, PhD, Pediatric Orthopedic Surgeon and Chief of Pediatric Orthopedic Department, Hospital Pequeno Principe and Hospital das Clinicas da UFPR, Curitiba, Brazil

DAVID A. SPIEGEL, MD, Assistant Professor of Orthopaedic Surgery, University of Pennsylvania School of Medicine; Division of Orthopaedic Surgery, Children's Hospital of Philadelphia, Philadelphia, Pennsylvania

DANIEL J. SUCATO, MD, MS, Staff Orthopedist, Texas Scottish Rite Hospital for Children; Associate Professor, Department of Orthopaedic Surgery, University of Texas at Southwestern Medical Center, Dallas, Texas

MAREK SYNDER, MD, PhD, Professor of Medicine, Clinic of Orthopaedics and Pediatric Orthopaedics; Head, Orthopaedic Department, Medical University of Lodz, Lodz, Poland

WON JOON YOO, MD, Assistant Professor, Department of Orthopedic Surgery, Seoul National University Hospital, Seoul, Korea

CONTENTS

Preface ix
James T. Guille

Growth and Development of the Child's Hip 119
Mark C. Lee and Craig P. Eberson

> The child's hip begins in intrauterine development as a condensation of mesoderm in the lower limb bud that rapidly differentiates to resemble the adult hip by eight weeks of life. The developmental instructions are transmitted through complicated cell signaling pathways. From eight weeks of development to adolescence, further growth of the hip is focused on differentiation and the establishment of the adult arterial supply. The postnatal growth of the child's hip is a product of concurrent acetabular and proximal femoral growth from their corresponding growth plates. Absence of appropriate contact between acetabulum and proximal femur yields an incongruent joint. Multiple disease processes may be understood in light of this growth process, including Legg-Calvé-Perthes disease and developmental dysplasia of the hip.

Evaluation of the Child Who Has Hip Pain 133
Steven L. Frick

> Evaluation of children who have hip pain can be a diagnostic challenge. This article reviews pertinent history taking, physical examination, laboratory testing, and imaging studies that assist in reaching a correct diagnosis. It also reviews the diagnostic categories that are important in formulating a differential diagnosis to frame clinical decision making.

Role of Ultrasound in the Diagnosis and Management of Developmental Dysplasia of the Hip: An International Perspective 141
Marek Synder, H. Theodore Harcke, and Marcin Domzalski

> Early diagnosis of developmental dysplasia of the hip is very important for proper treatment. Different ultrasound techniques have been used for early diagnosis of developmental dysplasia of the hip, but two of them are widely used in orthopedic practice: Graf's technique in Europe and Harcke's method in the United States. Our experience has led us to use an ultrasound technique that combines the two methods. Use of ultrasound has reduced the number of late-presenting cases, shortened treatment time, and decreased the number of surgical procedures of the hip joint in Poland.

Treatment of Developmental Dysplasia of the Hip After Walking Age With Open Reduction, Femoral Shortening, and Acetabular Osteotomy   149
Edilson Forlin, Luiz A. Munhoz da Cunha, and Daniel C. Figueiredo

> The one-stage surgical treatment for developmental dysplasia of the hip—consisting of open reduction, femoral shortening, and pelvic osteotomy—is a demanding procedure, one that is more challenging, technically, than a staged procedure. It can, however, be done safely and effectively, providing good conditions for proper development of the hip joint in the older child who has untreated developmental dysplasia of the hip.

Treatment of Late Dysplasia with Ganz Osteotomy   161
Daniel J. Sucato

> Following careful study, the Ganz periacetabular osteotomy was introduced in 1988 for the treatment of adolescent and adult hip dysplasia. It offers a powerful and versatile ability to reorient the acetabulum, restoring near-normal biomechanics, improving symptoms, and delaying or preventing osteoarthritis. This article outlines hip dysplasia and the biomechanical deficiencies, the assessment of patients who have hip dysplasia, and the technique of performing the osteotomy. The early and mid follow-up radiographic and clinical outcomes are reviewed and complications associated with the procedure are discussed.

Operative Reconstruction for Septic Arthritis of the Hip   173
In Ho Choi, Won Joon Yoo, Tae-Joon Cho, and Chin Youb Chung

> The long-term effects of initial treatment for infantile septic arthritis of the hip differ and depend on patient age, infecting organism, and timing and adequacy of surgical and pharmacologic treatment. Appropriate and timely reconstructive operations benefit hip growth and development by providing the best possible hip joint mechanics at skeletal maturity. Any surgical treatment for severe sequelae, however, must be regarded as a measure that temporarily improves clinical function and delays the more definitive procedures that are reserved for adult patients. This article summarizes the surgical modalities currently available to reduce and stabilize a damaged femoral head and neck and to reconstruct femoral–acetabular articulation.

Evaluation and Treatment of Hip Dysplasia in Cerebral Palsy   185
David A. Spiegel and John M. Flynn

> Hip problems, including progressive subluxation, dislocation, and pain, are common in patients with cerebral palsy, particularly those who are nonambulatory with a large degree of spasticity. Clinical and radiographic screening facilitates early detection, and surgery is indicated to prevent progressive dysplasia. Although an early soft tissue release may prevent progressive subluxation in a subset of cases, bony reconstructive surgery is indicated for patients with established bony deformity. Salvage procedures are recommended to treat chronic pain caused by established subluxation or dislocation.

Hip Disorders in Children Who Have Spinal Cord Injury   197
James J. McCarthy and Randal R. Betz

> Little has been written regarding the assessment and treatment of hip disorders in children who have underlying paralysis. Each year approximately 2000 people younger than 20 years of age suffer a spinal cord injury (SCI). This compares with a larger number of children who have other forms of neurologic disorders, such as myelodysplasia, which

affects approximately 6000 newborns annually in the United States, and for which there is a large body of literature describing the natural history and treatment of hip disorders in children who have myelodysplasia. This article focuses on hip disorders in children who have SCI, although there is clearly commonality in hip disorders that transcends many neurologic disorders.

Evaluation and Treatment of Hip Dysplasia in Charcot-Marie-Tooth Disease 203
Gilbert Chan, J. Richard Bowen, and S. Jay Kumar

The hip dysplasia seen in Charcot-Marie-Tooth disease is neuromuscular in nature. It usually presents in the second or third decade of life and is initially asymptomatic but may later present with pain and gait abnormalities. Treatment should be aimed at addressing the acetabular and femoral components of the dysplasia. Early recognition is essential to avoid serious morbidity associated with the condition.

Controversies in Slipped Capital Femoral Epiphysis 211
Randall T. Loder

Slipped capital femoral epiphysis (SCFE) is a common adolescent hip disorder. This article reviews the major controversies in SCFE as of the year 2005. These are (1) treatment of the unstable SCFE, (2) the role of osteotomy in the treatment of SCFE, (3) prophylactic fixation of the contralateral hip in children presenting with unilateral SCFE, and (4) methods of fixation in the very young child with SCFE.

Fractures of the Hip in Children 223
James H. Beaty

Fractures of the hip are uncommon in children, and their importance is related not to the frequency of the injury but to the frequency of complications. Many of these complications can be minimized or avoided by anatomic reduction and internal fixation. Open reduction frequently is necessary to obtain a stable, anatomic reduction. Regardless of the age of the child, stable fixation of the fracture must be given priority over preservation of the proximal femoral physis. The development of osteonecrosis, however, is most likely related to the severity of the initial injury and is largely unaffected by treatment of the fracture.

Hip Arthroscopy in Children and Adolescents 233
Mininder S. Kocher and Ben Lee

Hip arthroscopy has become an established procedure for certain indications in adults; however, experience in children and adolescents has been more limited. This article reviews the technique, indications, and results of hip arthroscopy in children and adolescents.

Index 241

FORTHCOMING ISSUES

July 2006
Musculoskeletal Imaging
Peter L. Munk, MD, CM, FRCPC, and
Bassam Masri, MD, *Guest Editors*

October 2006
Sexual Dimorphism in Musculoskeletal Health
Laura L. Tosi, MD,
Mary I. O'Connor, MD, and
Letha Griffin, MD, *Guest Editors*

April 2007
Vascularized Bone Grafting in Orthopedic Surgery
Alexander Y. Shin, MD, and
Steven L. Moran, MD, *Guest Editors*

RECENT ISSUES

January 2006
Oncology
Rakesh Donthineni, MD, *Guest Editor*

October 2005
The Treatment of Unicompartmental Arthritis of the Knee
Jack M. Bert, MD, *Guest Editor*

July 2005
Nonfusion Technology in Spinal Surgery
Russel C. Huang, MD, and
Rudolf Bertagnoli, MD, *Guest Editors*

VISIT THESE RELATED WEB SITES

Access your subscription at:
www.theclinics.com

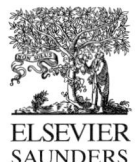
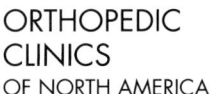

Preface
The Pediatric Hip

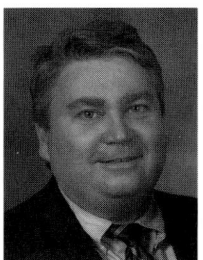

James T. Guille, MD
Guest Editor

It is daunting to be following in the footsteps of Dr. Mihran O. Tachdjian, who more than 25 years ago edited the last issue of the *Orthopedic Clinics of North America* devoted to the pediatric hip. It is amazing to look back upon that issue and see the advances we have made in our basic understanding of the pathophysiology of the various conditions, as well as their management. When outlining this issue, I purposefully did not read the table of contents from Dr. Tachdjian's work. Instead, I wanted to include what I thought would be practical articles pertinent for today's practicing pediatric orthopedist. I was then pleased to find that I had overlapped in only three areas: cerebral palsy, developmental dysplasia of the hip (DDH), and septic arthritis. Dr. Tachdjian's issue included contributions from authors in North America, as well as Scotland and Australia. We are honored to have not only our North American contributors, but also authors from Korea, Brazil, and Poland.

Twenty-five years ago, Dr. Eberson would not have had the advancements in basic science to have written his excellent article on "Growth and Development of the Child's Hip." Dr. Synder and his associates have outlined their algorithm for the "Role of Ultrasound in the Diagnosis and Management of Developmental Dysplasia of the Hip," a technique that was in its infancy in 1980. Dr. Forlin and colleagues share with us their experience in treating DDH in the older child with open reduction, femoral shortening, and pelvic osteotomy, a treatment few surgeons would have tackled in the past. In the previous issue, Dr. John Handelsman wrote on the role of Chiari osteotomy in the older child with DDH; in this issue, Dr. Sucato writes on the newer Ganz osteotomy. One has to wonder what new, yet-unconceived osteotomy will be written about in 2031. Drs. McCarthy and Betz tell us their experience with hip problems in patients with spinal cord injury, and Dr. Kumar and associates detail the nuances about the hip in patients with Charcot-Marie-Tooth disease. In keeping with the explosion of interest in the area of minimally invasive surgery, Dr. Kocher writes on the innovation of hip arthroscopy in children.

It is my hope that the knowledge gleaned from this issue of the *Orthopedic Clinics of North America* not only helps us treat the routine pediatric hip conditions that we see every week, but also those that we may see only once a year. Finally, I would be remiss if I did not thank the contributors of this issue in addition to my mentors in the field, Drs. Richard Bowen, Jay Kumar, and Dean MacEwen.

James T. Guille, MD
Shriners Hospital for Children
3551 North Broad Street
Philadelphia, PA 19140, USA
E-mail address: jguille@shrinenet.org

Growth and Development of the Child's Hip

Mark C. Lee, MD[a], Craig P. Eberson, MD[b],*

[a]Brown Medical School, Department of Orthopaedics, Rhode Island Hospital, 593 Eddy Street, Providence, RI 02903, USA
[b]Brown Medical School, Department of Orthopaedics, Hasbro Children's Hospital, Providence, Rhode Island, USA

The normal child's hip is the result of an intricate balance between a growing acetabulum, a growing proximal femur, and the vasculature that accommodates to the bony changes. The program for hip development begins with a genetic template actuated by a cascade of cell signaling factors. Within the outline provided by the genetic code, embryonic, fetal, and childhood development of the hip continue while changing to a variety of environmental and biologic factors.

Understanding the sequential steps of the hip's development, along with the growth of its blood supply, is critical to elucidate the pathobiologic mechanisms of hip disease and deformity in the child. Even more critical is the ability to devise and apply rational treatments for pediatric orthopedic diseases that can take advantage of known growth mechanisms. This article discusses the current knowledge of the growth of the normal child's hip from the embryo to adolescence. Abnormal growth of the pediatric hip is then examined through an analysis of two common disease processes and their treatments.

Normal development of the child's hip

Prenatal cellular development

Prenatal human development is separated into an embryonic stage and a fetal stage. The embryonic stage begins when the oocyte is fertilized and ends at approximately 8 weeks postfertilization. During the first three weeks of the embryonic stage, the primitive ectoderm, mesoderm, and endoderm germ layers are formed in the embryonic disc. It is during the fourth to the eighth weeks of development that the majority of joint differentiation is completed [1]. The fetal stage encompasses the period from the eighth week of life to birth. During this period, the limbs and joints undergo growth and maturation in relative proportions and pre-established spatial orientations [1].

Limb formation begins at 4 weeks of development with protrusions of the ventro–lateral wall of the embryo, termed limb buds. The upper limb buds usually appear 2 to 3 days earlier than the lower. Each limb bud consists of an outer ectoderm shell, from which skin, nails, and hair develop, and an inner cellular mass of mesoderm, from which bone, cartilage, muscle, tendon, and the synovial joints arise.

By the sixth week of intrauterine life, the lower limb buds have elongated and now include paddle-like ends termed foot plates (Fig. 1). Vigorous cell multiplication and differentiation occur in the substance of the limb bud. Primitive chondroblasts condense at the proximal, central, and distal ends of the cellular femur template. The club-shaped cartilage model of the future femur follows from these centers through successive chondrification of the precursor cells and fusion of the chondrification centers [1].

The acetabulum begins at 6 weeks as a shallow depression proximal to the head of the femur and is formed by the differentiating precursor cells of the future ilium, ischium, and pubis (Fig. 2). The cartilage model of the acetabulum is formed concurrently with the cartilage model of the pelvic components. Condensations of cartilage cells appear first in the primitive ilium, and then the pubis, and finally the ischium. Chondrification proceeds from these

* Corresponding author. Rhode Island Hospital Medical Office Center, 2 Dudley Street, Providence, RI 02905.
E-mail address: ceberson@lifespan.org (C.P. Eberson).

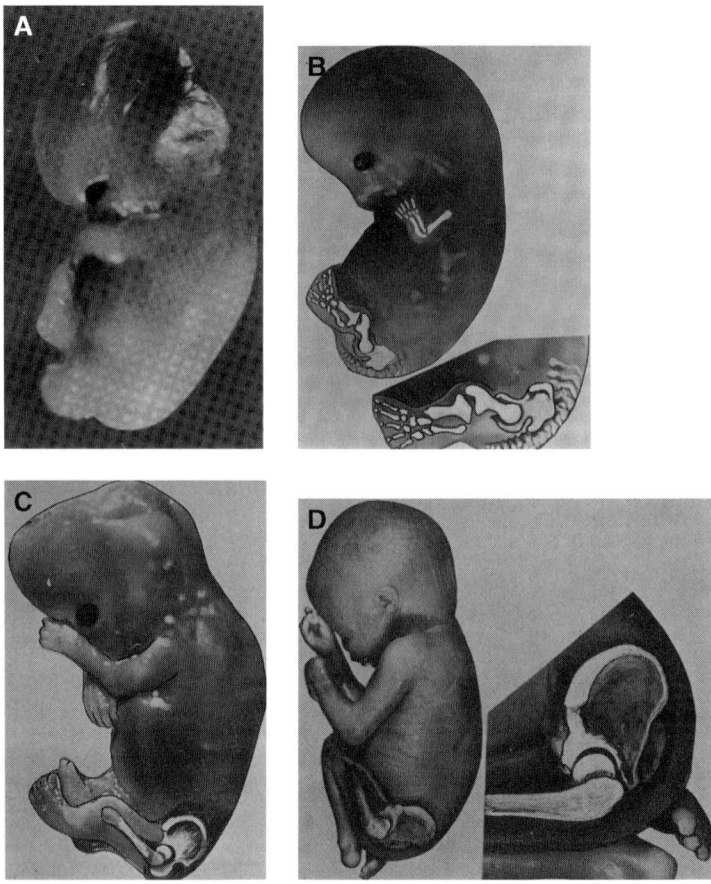

Fig. 1. (*A*) Viewed macroscopically, at the age of 6 weeks, the embryo is 1 cm in size and the limb buds have begun the process of differentiation. Hand and foot plates are visible. (*B*) At the age of 8 weeks, there has been further differentiation of limb buds such that the hip, knee, ankle, and feet are well-formed structures. (*C*) At the age of 11 weeks, there has been a rapid differentiation of the hip joint; and the infantile configuration of the femoral head and acetabulum is now present. (*D*) At the age of 16 weeks, the fetus now measures 100 cm. The lower extremities lie in a position of stability for the fetal hip joint, specifically flexion, adduction, and external rotation. (*Adapted from* Watanabe RS. Embryology of the human hip. Clin Orthop 1974;98:8,12,14,20; with permission.)

centers toward each other until fusion occurs. The chondrification centers fuse quickly, with the ilium and ischium joining first, followed by the ilium and the pubis. The pubis and ischium centers are the last to fuse, closing during the seventh week, and leave a small opening laterally, corresponding to the apex of the developing acetabular fossa [2]. Note that differentiation of the acetabulum, especially the ilium, lags behind that of the femoral head and shaft at all stages.

By the seventh week of gestation, the cartilaginous model for both the femur and acetabulum are complete. The mass of primitive cells between the femoral and acetabular cartilage models now undergo apoptosis to yield a fluid-filled cleft, the beginning of the future hip joint [2]. Theoretically, this stage is the earliest time in development during which a hip dislocation may occur [2].

By the eighth week of development, at the transition from the embryo stage to the fetal stage, the primary ossification center of the femur now appears in its shaft. Ossification proceeds proximally and distally from this center. The soft tissue components of the hip have begun to take shape also. A grouping of cells adjacent to the femoral head identifies the future site of the ligamentum teres and is continuous with the condensation of cells marking the future transverse acetabular ligament inferiorly. The ligamentum teres is defined as the joint space expands and is seen to attach to the medial border of the acetabular fossa, separating from the transverse

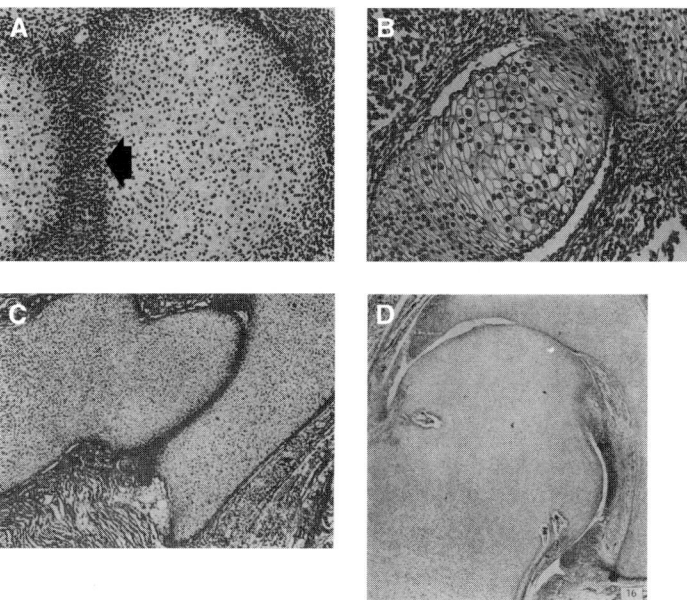

Fig. 2. (*A*) Viewed microscopically, at 4 weeks, condensation of the cells in the interval between the primitive femoral head and the acetabulum occurs to form the hip joint. (*B*) At 7 weeks, the femoral head has a spherical contour; and the acetabulum develops rapidly around it. Note the beginning of a joint cavity at this stage. (*C*) At 8 weeks, the early cartilage model of the acetabulum and femoral head has begun to form. The majority of hip structures, including the labrum, are identifiable at this stage. (*D*) At 11 to 14 weeks, blood vessels are observed to enter through the small lacunae hollowed out of the head and neck. The labrum along the periphery of the acetabulum and the ligamentum teres of the femur are visible. (*A–C adapted from* Watanabe RS. Embryology of the human hip. Clin Orthop 1974;98:10,11; with permission, and *D adapted from* Strayer Jr LM. Embryology of the human hip joint. Clin Orthop 1971;74:236; with permission.)

acetabular ligament to lie behind it. The acetabular labrum is observed at 6 weeks as a condensation of cells lying along the periphery of the developing acetabulum that rides the enlarging rim of the ilium, ischium, and pubis out over the femoral head. By the eighth week, it has begun to assume its triangular configuration in coronal section. The joint capsule and synovia may be distinguished at 8 weeks as a layer of cells lying under the muscular primordia and over the acetabular labrum, joining the perichondrium of the femur below.

Although hip differentiation continues until approximately 20 weeks of development, the major anatomic structures of the hip are identifiable microscopically by the eighth week. Passage into the fetal stage at this point is characterized by a shift from differentiation to growth and maturation of the hip. By 11 weeks, all portions of the hip are visible macroscopically, and the infantile configuration of the hip joint is achieved. The femoral head is formed fully with spherical contour, short femoral neck, and a primitive greater trochanter (see Fig. 2D). A well-defined capsule is present, as are the acetabular labrum and transverse ligament. The hip can be actively dislocated at this time.

At 16 weeks, the ossification of the femur is complete up to the level of the lesser trochanter. The primary centers of ossification have appeared in the ilium, ischium, and pubis, although the acetabular ossification centers do not appear until adolescence [2]. The hip joint space is now completely formed, and the articular surfaces are covered with mature hyaline cartilage. All of the muscle structures are mature, and active motion of the extremities can now be observed.

Limb position, femoral anteversion, and neck–shaft angle

At 4 weeks, the embryo has begun to show slight flexion at the knee [2]. During the eighth week of development, the lower limb begins rotating internally to direct the flexed knee anteriorly and completes the rotation by the end of the embryonic stage. At 11 weeks, the hip and knee are flexed and the leg is adducted. By 16 weeks, further flexion occurs at the hip and knee; and the left leg is noted to slightly overlap the right leg. With continued growth and accommodation of the developing fetus to a closed space, further flexion of the fetal hip and knee occur until the fetal position is assumed [2].

Femoral anteversion is first able to be discerned at 11 weeks and measures 5° to 10°. Jouve and colleagues [3] studied 87 femurs from 44 formalin-preserved fetuses and demonstrated a wide variability in anteversion position at each fetal age, especially during the first half of fetal life, but noted an increase with increasing fetal age, measuring on average 45° at 36 weeks. Femoral anteversion then decreases in postnatal development. Fabry and colleagues [4] studied 432 healthy children (864 hips) and developed a normal baseline of femoral anteversion at each age from 1 to 16 years. The mean angle of femoral anteversion was 31.1° at age 1 year, decreasing to 15.4° by age 16 years [4].

Neck–shaft angle in fetal development appears to decrease with fetal age, ranging from approximately 145° at 15 weeks to 130° at 36 weeks [3]. Following birth, the neck–shaft angle progressively decreases with age. Zippel [5] studied 400 children (800 hips) and developed a normal baseline of neck–shaft angle at each age from 1 to 20 years. The mean neck–shaft angle at age 1 year was 136.2°, whereas at age 18 years, the value dropped to 127.3°.

The mechanism for femoral anteversion and neck–shaft angle formation in the fetal period remains elusive. Initial speculation that anteversion results from the normal internal rotation of the lower limb during development is countered by the observation that femoral anteversion changes long after the completion of limb rotation. Watanabe [2] noted that excessive internal rotation or external rotation of the fetal limb in a specimen was associated with excessive femoral anteversion or retroversion, respectively. He theorized that the proximal femur position is likely related to the muscular forces that act on the hip during prenatal development.

The argument that muscular forces across the hip joint influence femoral anteversion and neck–shaft angle is more cogent in the postnatal hip. In a cross-sectional study of 267 hips in 147 patients who had cerebral palsy between the ages of 2 and 18 years, Bobroff and colleagues [6] demonstrated radiographically that femoral anteversion remained relatively constant at each postpartum age in the cerebral palsy group, whereas it decreased in the historical control group. Further, patients who had cerebral palsy were noted to have a markedly increased neck–shaft angle at each age as compared with historical controls. The difference is presumably the result of muscle spasticity and soft tissue contracture about the hips of patients who have cerebral palsy.

Cell signaling in intrauterine joint development

The formation of the joint is a complicated sequence of cellular events that involves the creation of mesenchymal aggregates, the condensation of mesenchymal precursors on either side of the joint with the formation of a less dense interzone, and cavitation of the interzone to form the future joint space. The ossification of the cartilage anlage of the long bone occurs simultaneously. Advances in molecular techniques have allowed the bone morphogenetic proteins (BMPs), a family of secreted cell-signaling molecules with key roles in development, to be identified as the crucial components of joint formation. An understanding of the synergistic and antagonistic roles of the myriad known signals for ordered joint formation remains obscure, however.

Growth and differentiation factor 5 (GDF-5) is a much-studied BMP necessary for proper joint development. GDF-5 is localized as stripes at the future sites of joints in mouse embryos [7,8]. GDF-5 is expressed in almost all of the developing joints of the limb from early stages of cellular condensation to joint cavitation [9,10]. When creating a null mutation of GDF-5 in mice, a brachypodism (short-limbed mutant) phenotype results where the appendicular skeleton is shortened and the formation of approximately 30% of the joints of the limb is disrupted [9]. The relevance of GDF-5 to human joint development is clear when considering the skeletal dysplasias that result from mutations in the human homologue CDMP1, including Hunter-Thompson-type acromesomelic chondroplasia, autosomal dominant brachydactyly type C, and Grebe-type chondrodysplasia [11–13].

A solution to the message for joint formation lies not in defining the function of the various molecular signals, but rather in their complex interaction. Examination of the BMP inhibiting protein noggin exemplifies this complexity. In mice homozygous for the noggin loss of function allele, a single cartilaginous limb element results with no joint formation (Fig. 3) [8]. The implication is that unchecked BMP activity disturbs the patterning of the joint. The concept is reinforced by examining the activity of BMP-7, which has been shown to be highly expressed in the perichondrial cells of the avian embryo surrounding condensing chondrocytes and promotes cartilage formation [7]. BMP-7 is absent in the cell

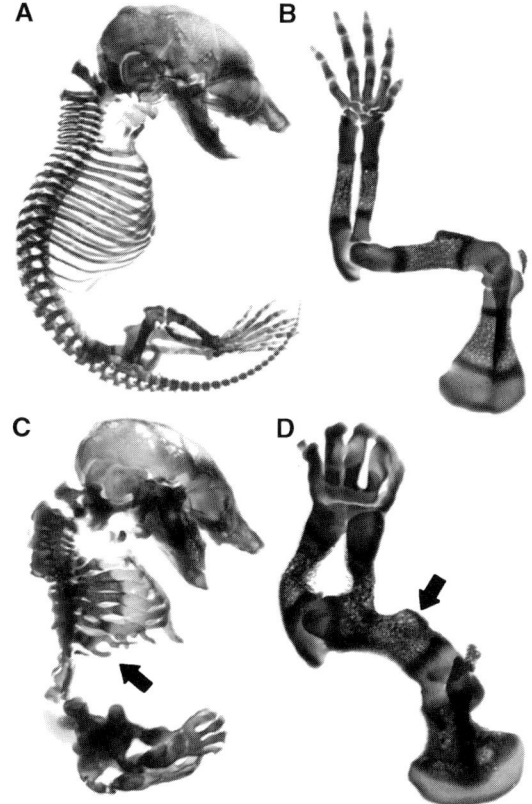

Fig. 3. Skeletal abnormalities in noggin homozygous mouse mutants. Skeletons, with forelimbs removed, from wild-type (*A*) and mutant (*C*) embryos 18.5 days postcoitum were stained blue for nonmineralized cartilage and red for mineralized cartilage and bone. The forelimbs are shown in (*B*) and (*D*), respectively. In (*C*), the solid arrow points to multiple rib deformities and fusions. Note the failure of formation of the spine, knee, ankle, hindfoot, and midfoot. In (*D*), the solid arrow points to continuous ossification from the radius to humerus. Note the failure of formation of elbow and carpus. (*Adapted from* Brunet LJ, McMahon JA, McMahon AP, et al. Noggin, cartilage morphogenesis, and joint formation in the mammalian skeleton. Science 1998; 280(5368):1456; with permission.)

condensations marking the future joints. When beads secreting BMP-7 are implanted into these condensations, joint formation is inhibited [7]. The mechanisms that clear BMP-7 expression at the sites of joint development are therefore crucial for normal joint development.

The temporal expression of various protein elements further complicates the understanding of cellular joint morphogenesis. Each stage of development may be thought to contain a specific cell-signaling milieu. The action of each signal does not occur in a vacuum, but is modified by the presence of other signals. To exemplify, BMPs can induce death or differentiation depending on the stage of development. Application of excessive BMP-2 or BMP-7 beads to the developing chick limb bud before mesenchyme condensation induces apoptosis and a subsequent loss of skeletal elements [7]. If the BMP-2 and BMP-7 beads are applied two days later, cartilage formation is induced and the limbs resemble those of noggin mutants. BMP-2 and BMP-7 activity is changed completely by other proteins either present or absent at different times of development. This "context dependency" of signal action is an important general principle in the development of the vertebrate limb and provides an underpinning for understanding the role of various molecules [14].

Postnatal development of the child's hip

Acetabular development

At birth, the acetabular cartilage complex consists of the saucer-shaped acetabular cartilage laterally and the Y-shaped triradiate cartilage medially (Fig. 4). These two components of the acetabular cartilage complex are continuous, and their coordinated growth results in the final acetabular shape [15]. Eventually the triradiate cartilage will form the nonarticular medial wall of the acetabulum; and the acetabular cartilage will form the cup-shaped rim of the acetabulum.

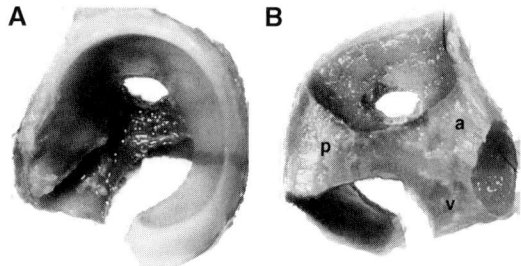

Fig. 4. Lateral view (*A*) and medial view (*B*) of the normal acetabular cartilage complex of a one-day-old infant. The ilium, ischium, and pubis have been removed with a curette. The lateral view shows the cup-shaped acetabulum, and the medial view shows the three flanges of the triradiate cartilage. The anterior flange (*a*) is located between the ilium and pubis and is slanted superiorly; the posterior flange (*p*) is horizontal and located between the ilium and ischium; the vertical flange (*v*) is located between the pubis and ischium. (*Adapted from* Ponseti IV. Growth and development of the acetabulum in the normal child. Anatomical, histological, and roentgenographic studies. J Bone Joint Surg Am 1978;60(5):576; with permission.)

The acetabular cartilage complex is composed of mostly hyaline cartilage. The hyaline cartilage is covered by growth plate cartilage at all areas where it lies adjacent to the bony pelvis and by articular cartilage at all the points of contact with the femoral head. The labrum forms the outer margin of the acetabulum, increasing its relative depth, and is made of fibrocartilage.

The acetabular cartilage complex is an epiphysis and develops in much the same way as the iliac crest and the epiphysis of long bones with the appearance of secondary ossification centers. Three main acetabular ossification centers develop in the acetabular cartilage in humans. The os acetabuli is the largest and forms in the cartilage contributed by the pubis. It is the functional epiphysis of the pubis, as it is separated from the pubis by a growth plate. The os acetabuli initially occupies the anterior part of the acetabular floor and eventually forms the anterior wall of the acetabulum. The iliac acetabular cartilage center forms the superior acetabular bone and joint surface. The ischial acetabular center, the smallest of the three, develops to form the posterior acetabulum. All ossification centers appear by 8 to 9 years of age and fuse by 17 to 18 years of age. Since most of the acetabular shape is determined by 8 years, this age is important for prognosis in many pediatric hip disorders [16,17].

The growth of acetabular height and width depends on the interstitial growth of the triradiate cartilage. Growth in depth and the construction of the final acetabular shape, however, heavily depends on the interaction with a spherical femoral head. When the femoral heads in growing rats were excised or dislocated, Harrison [18] found that the acetabular socket failed to develop in depth and there was atrophy and degeneration of the articular cartilage, while the triradiate cartilage remained histologically normal. The acetabulum requires the spherical femoral head as a template about which it forms. In fact, the condition of proximal focal femoral deficiency punctuates the interplay between the developing femoral head and the developing acetabulum. Presence in part of the proximal femur allows development of an acetabulum. Complete absence of the proximal femur yields an absent acetabulum [1].

Proximal femoral development

The ossification of the cartilaginous femoral shaft proceeds proximally during the fetal stage to reach the greater trochanter and femoral neck at birth. The cartilage template of the proximal femur that has not

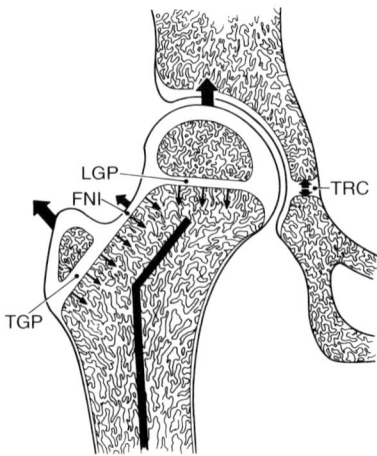

Fig. 5. Development of the hip during infancy and childhood occurs by proliferation of growth cartilage (unshaded) of the acetabulum and the proximal femur. The acetabulum grows appositionally through growth of the articular cartilage and interstitially through growth of the triradiate cartilage (TRC). The head of the femur and greater trochanter enlarge by appositional growth. The three growth zones of the proximal femur are: the longitudinal growth plate (LGP), the trochanteric growth plate (TGP) and the femoral neck isthmus (FNI). (*Adapted from* Siffert RS. Patterns of deformity of the developing hip. Clin Orthop Relat Res 1981; Oct(160):16; with permission.)

been replaced by bone defines three growth plates: the longitudinal growth plate of the neck (LGP), the greater trochanteric growth plate (TGP), and the femoral neck isthmus (FNI) [19] (Fig. 5). These three growth plates work concurrently to support the longitudinal growth of the femur and to develop the shape of the proximal femur. Of note, the growth plate of the lesser trochanter and its iliopsoas attachment are poorly studied but do not appear to influence the growth of the proximal or distal femur.

The LGP anatomically lies within the head of the femur during infancy and initially contributes to the maintenance of its sphericity. As the neck elongates, the geographic center of the head moves proximally until the LGP achieves its final position at the junction of the femoral head and neck. The LGP grows proximally and medially, contributing to the longitudinal growth of the femur and neck, as well as to the lateral width of the femoral neck.

The TGP lies at the base of the cartilage template of the greater trochanter. Like the LGP, it contributes mainly to the longitudinal growth of the proximal femur and to the lateral width of the femoral neck. Similarities emerge when examining the relationship of the greater trochanter and the femoral head to their respective proximal femoral growth plates. Both the greater trochanter and femoral head enlarge through appositional growth of their cartilage precursors with subsequent ossification; however, their final positions in space relative to the femur and each other are determined by the proximal femoral growth plates upon which they rest. The greater trochanter is forced proximally and laterally by the TGP, and the femoral head is forced proximally and medially by the LGP.

The FNI is a small cartilage isthmus spared by ossification that connects the trochanteric and femoral neck plates along the lateral border of the femoral neck. The FNI dynamically contributes to the lateral width of the neck, keeping pace with the TGP and LGP. Since no growth in femoral neck width occurs along the medial border of the neck, the varus and valgus angulation of the neck is controlled by the contributions to the lateral growth of the neck by the three growth plates.

The dynamic relationship of the LGP, TGP, and FNI can be examined in terms of growth vectors. The TGP and FNI have growth vectors that are oriented divergently with respect to the LGP. All three growth plates are at an angle relative to the long axis of the femoral shaft. Concurrent function of the three growth plates yields not only growth along their respective axis, but also a common vector of growth directed along the axis of the femoral shaft. A disturbance in any one of these growth plates can lead to angular abnormalities of the proximal femur. Further, growth rates may be controlled by altering the position of the growth plate relative to the femoral shaft. For example, during infancy and childhood, the LGP is relatively horizontal and perpendicular to the long axis of the femur. As the TGP and FNI growth rates increase toward adolescence, the LGP begins to tip medially, allowing for a constant rate of longitudinal growth and allowing a more medially directed vector to balance proximal growth of the femoral neck. A disruption of this normal growth pattern is seen in Ogden type II avascular necrosis, where the FNI and lateral aspect of the LGP suffer a vascular insult. The femoral head tips into a valgus position as growth stops along the lateral aspect of the LGP and continues along the medial.

Just as a located femoral head is necessary for acetabular development, it is also necessary for correct femoral head development. The contact pressures exerted on the femoral head cartilage by the tight-fitting acetabulum result in its spherical appositional growth, as increasing pressure inhibits growth. Likewise, the pressure exerted by the femoral head on the acetabulum is critical to the achievement of the complementary acetabular shape. Proximal femur and acetabulum development are inextricably linked to achieve the end goal of a congruent joint.

Development of the arterial supply to the child's hip

The origin of the arterial organization of the child's hip may be divided into the development of the vessels along the femoral and acetabular sides. The arterial supply to the proximal femur begins its development with the appearance of the primary ossification center in the femoral shaft during the eighth week of development. Capillaries break through the periosteum at the middle third of the femoral shaft cartilage template, at the level of the nutrient artery in the adult femur, and carry fibroblastic and hematopoeitic cells into the marrow. For many weeks in development, it is the only intraosseous blood supply in the entire femur [1]. By 12 to14 weeks of development, a ring of vessels has begun to form around the neck of the femur, consisting of the future medial and lateral circumflex vessels, the obturator, and the superior and inferior gluteal vessels. At this point, blood vessels connected to this ring have invaded the cartilage model of the head and neck of the femur; and capillary tufts form along the neck of the femur at the future site of the retinacular vessels.

The entry of blood vessels into the acetabulum occurs just after the entry of blood vessels into the head and neck of the femur during weeks 12 to14 of development [1]. However, the ligamentum teres and the fibrofatty tissue filling the acetabular fossa, known as the Haversian gland or the pulvinar, have evidence of capillary invasion by 8 weeks. The significance of the vasculature at these two sites for further growth and development of the hip is questionable. Strayer [1] notes that only one of seven large fetuses examined showed vessels entering the femoral head from the ligamentum teres and that vessels from the ligamentum teres invade the head only after ossification is well under way. No anastomosis with the distal arterial terminals in the femoral head was observed until around age 15, when ossification of the head is nearly complete [20]. The findings suggest that the artery of the ligamentum teres does not offer a significant contribution to the blood supply of the developing femoral head. In fact, removal of the ligamentum teres during open reduction of a dysplastic hip does not result in adverse growth consequences.

The organization of the blood supply to the proximal end of the femur established during pre-natal development endures throughout the growth of the child. Chung's perfusion study [20] of 150 proximal

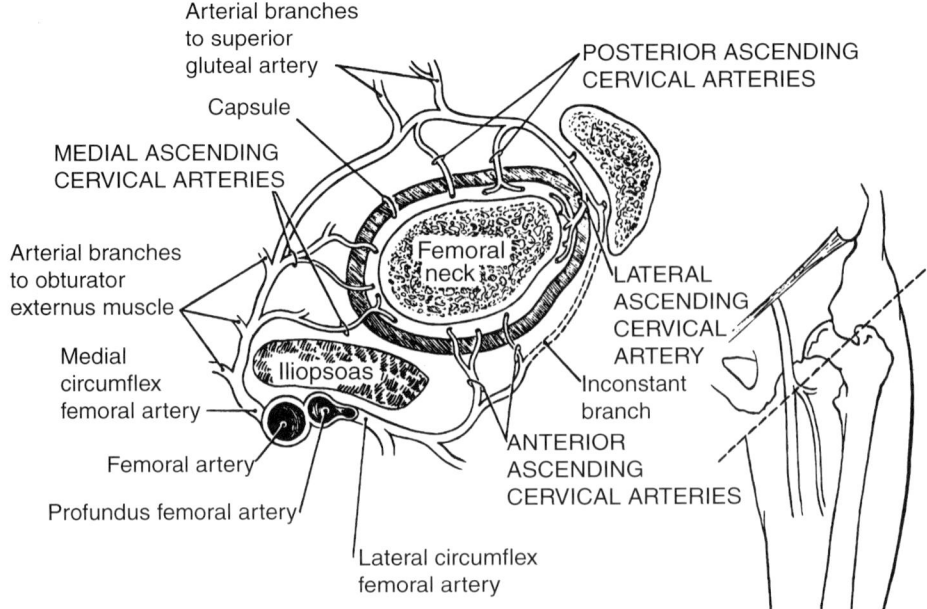

Fig. 6. Cross-section of proximal part of the left femur at the base of the neck, showing the extracapsular arterial ring. Broken lines indicate inconstant connections between anterior and lateral ascending cervical arteries. The lateral ascending cervical artery branches after traversing the capsule. In young children, it lies in the narrow space between the femoral neck and greater trochanter. (*Adapted from* Chung SM. The arterial supply of the developing proximal end of the human femur. J Bone Joint Surg Am 1976;58(7):964; with permission.)

femurs from autopsied fetuses and children aged 26 weeks to 14 years demonstrated that the vessel configuration largely maintains the final adult anatomy during development.

The proximal femur arterial supply in a growing child consists of (1) an extracapsular arterial ring (Fig. 6), (2) intracapsular ascending cervical arteries (Figs. 7–9), and (3) an intracapsular subsynovial ring (Fig. 10). The extracapsular arterial ring rests at the base of the femoral neck and is formed by the union of branches from the medial and lateral circumflex arteries. From the extracapsular ring, thin ascending cervical or retinacular vessels pierce the hip capsule and travel in a subsynovial, intra-articular location along the femoral neck toward the head. Four groups of such vessels are identified and named based on anatomic location relative to the femoral neck: lateral, posterior, medial, and anterior. Branches from the ascending cervical arteries pierce the neck of the femur and travel distally to the metaphysis to follow one of three fates. First, these branches may turn laterally and supply the greater trochanter. Second, they may anastomose with the ascending nutrient vessels from the femoral shaft. Finally, they may turn medially and supply the femoral neck.

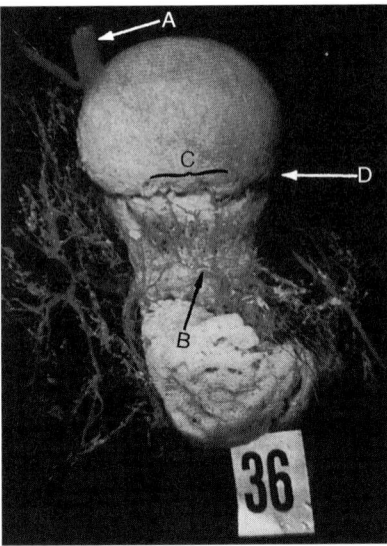

Fig. 7. Superolateral view of proximal part of the left femur from a 14.67-year-old boy perfused with Baton's medium. The femoral artery (*A*), extracapsular ring (*B*), ascending lateral cervical arteries (*C*), and physeal plate (*D*) are demonstrated. (*Adapted from* Chung SM. The arterial supply of the developing proximal end of the human femur. J Bone Joint Surg Am 1976;58(7):964; with permission.)

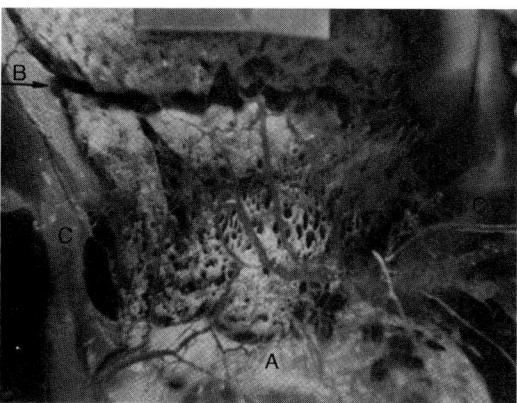

Fig. 8. Close-up of the same specimen as shown in Fig. 7 detailing the lateral ascending cervical arteries. Note the capillaries to the greater trochanter (A). The physeal plate (B) and the capsule (C) are visible as well. (*Adapted from* Chung SM. The arterial supply of the developing proximal end of the human femur. J Bone Joint Surg Am 1976;58(7):964; with permission.)

The ascending cervical vessels unite more proximally at the junction of the femoral neck and the articular cartilage of the head to form an intra-articular subsynovial arterial ring anastomosis. This ring is sometimes incomplete, more often in males,

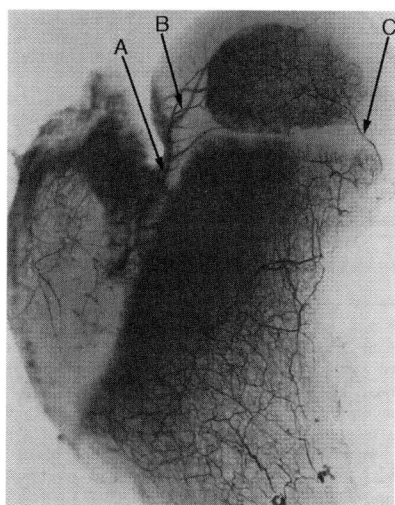

Fig. 9. Anterior half of proximal part of the right femur, perfused with barium sulfate and then divided in the coronal plane, from a 40-month-old white boy. The lateral ascending cervical artery (A) and the epiphyseal branches of the lateral (B) and medial (C) ascending cervical arteries are seen to pass through the perichondrial ring and not the physeal plate. (*Adapted from* Chung SM. The arterial supply of the developing proximal end of the human femur. J Bone Joint Surg Am 1976;58(7):964; with permission.)

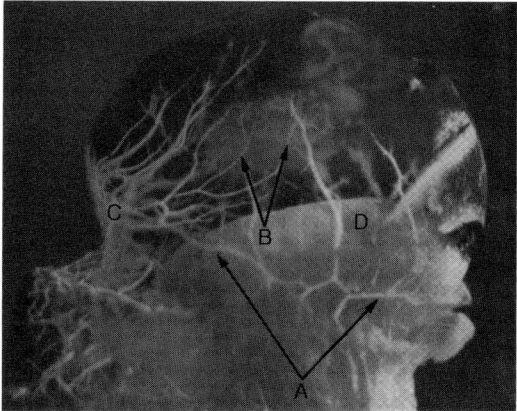

Fig. 10. Anterior view of the right femoral neck, perfused with barium sulfate, from a 9-month-old girl. The intracapsular subsynovial ring (A) is visualized. Multiple vessels are seen to supply the ossification center (B). Numerous branches of the lateral ascending cervical arteries (C) are seen to skirt the edge of the epiphysis and do not cross through the metaphysis (D). (*Adapted from* Chung SM. The arterial supply of the developing proximal end of the human femur. J Bone Joint Surg Am 1976;58(7):967; with permission.)

and is typically more robust on the medial and lateral surfaces of the femoral neck than the anterior and posterior [20]. From here, epiphyseal and metaphyseal branches ensue. The epiphyseal branches cross the physeal plate by skirting the perichondrial ring superficially and then enter the cartilage of the developing femoral head. The metaphyseal branches pierce the femoral neck and travel distally.

It is commonly assumed that the clinical importance of the pelvic and acetabular blood supply may be far less than that of the proximal femur, given the wide range of intraosseous and extraosseous anastomosis. Since the adult blood supply is established by the postnatal course, an understanding of the configuration allows the surgeon to avoid at least a theoretic incidence of acetabular avascular necrosis and growth arrest during pelvic osteotomy. The configuration of the vessels about the acetabulum may be understood if the acetabulum is divided into sectors as in the face of a clock (Fig. 11). At approximately 10 o'clock to 4 o'clock, branches of the superior gluteal artery supply the acetabular dome; at 4 o'clock to 8 o'clock, the posterior branch of the obturator extends nutrient arteries to the inferior acetabular bone; at 8 o'clock to 10 o'clock, a branch of inferior gluteal artery provides nutrient acetabular branches [22]. Despite the division into sectors, a rich extraosseous and intraosseous anastomosis exists between

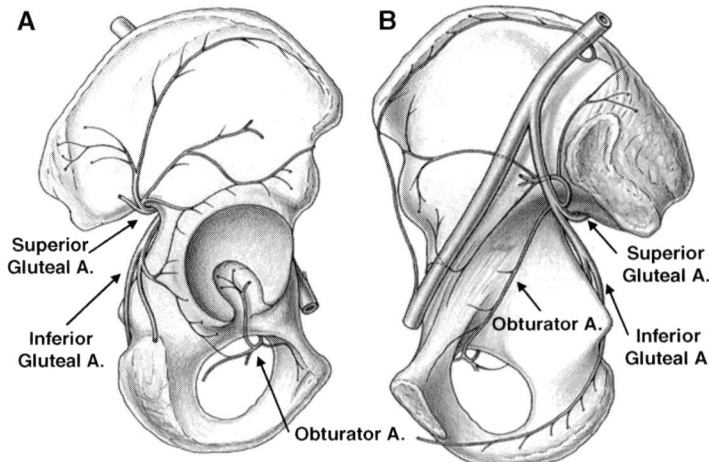

Fig. 11. Lateral (*A*) and medial (*B*) views of the right acetabulum with its associated vascular supply. Note the clockwise arrangement of the superior gluteal artery, obturator artery, and inferior gluteal artery contributions to the acetabulum. (*Adapted from* Beck, et al. The acetabular blood supply: implications for periacetabular osteotomies. Surg Radiol Anat 2003;25:365; with permission.)

these vessels. The redundancy of the vascular supply may explain why avascular necrosis of the acetabulum is rare after pelvic osteotomy, even when done at a young age. For example, bilateral pelvic osteotomies for bladder extrophy repair rarely have untoward results for acetabular growth.

The configuration of the blood vessels about the proximal femur in the child brings to light two important differences between the vascular anatomy of the child and the adult hip. One difference is the presence of a growth plate. From birth to the time of physeal plate closure, the plate is a vascular barrier and no vessels cross it. The ascending cervical vessels access the femoral head by coursing along the perimeter of the growth plate. Note that an extraosseous anastomosis still exists between the intraosseous microcirculation of the head and neck through the subsynovial arterial ring. After physeal plate closure, the metaphyseal vessels penetrate into the epiphysis, and the vascular systems communicate along intraosseous routes [21].

Second, when the cervical arteries penetrated into the cartilaginous femoral head during growth, independent vascular territories were initially defined. In later growth, these territories appear to coalesce into a large anastomotic network. It is speculated that this network is not complete, and occlusion of specific ascending arteries may cause necrosis of previously defined autonomous vascular zones.

Finally, the medial circumflex artery and its terminal end, the lateral portion of the extracapsular arterial ring, provide the majority of the blood supply to the femoral head, neck and greater trochanter [20]. As the child grows, the contribution of the medial circumflex artery assumes greater significance, because the number of cervical arteries contributed by the lateral circumflex artery decrease in development. Chung [20] found an approximately 50% reduction in the number of vessels along the anterior and medial aspect of the femoral neck when comparing children from 0 to 2 years of age and children from 3 to 10 years of age. The number of lateral and posterior ascending cervical arteries, derived from the medial circumflex branch, remained constant. Lauritzen [23] also confirmed that by age 10 the lateral retinacular arteries begin to dominate the blood supply to the head and neck of the femur.

Abnormal development of the child's hip

Developmental dysplasia of the hip

Developmental dysplasia of the hip (DDH) is a disease process that encompasses a spectrum of anatomic hip abnormalities in the newborn ranging from mild dysplastic acetabular change to complete teratologic (antenatal) dislocation. The incidence of DDH is reported as 1 to 1.5 per 1000 live births, but 1 out of 100 newborns may have some evidence of "hip instability" [24].

The causes of DDH are multifactorial, including both genetic and mechanical factors. Genetic factors are illustrated by the increased incidence of the disease in patients of female gender, a positive family history, or a particular ethnic background, such as North American Indian and Laplander. Mechanical factors are illustrated by the increased risk in patients who experienced breech presentation, oligohydramnios, or other "crowding" conditions.

Pivotal to determining etiology is whether or not the acetabular dysplasia characteristic of the disease is a result of primary abnormal acetabular development or secondary to intrauterine hip subluxation or dislocation. A primary etiology would suggest a genetic basis for the disease, implicating a failure in cell-signaling pathways and an intrinsic error in hip growth and development. Acetabular dysplasia secondary to hip subluxation would then support mechanical theories as the primary cause of DDH. In this case, as noted previously, the dislocation may not occur until the joint cavity opens at the seventh week of development and may then result from the failure to keep the head pointed at the acetabulum as a result of extrafetal mechanical pressures favoring dislocation. Dislocation may then occur through the posterior–inferior acetabulum, at the site of the future transverse ligament, the weakest point in the labral structure [1]. The deficiency posteriorly and inferiorly corresponds to the postnatal anatomic abnormality in the hip. Since acetabular depth in the fetus is directly correlated with head size, the fetal acetabulum also becomes shallow [25].

Late diagnosis of DDH and its associated anatomic abnormalities illustrates many of the mechanical growth principles of the child's hip and the necessary interaction between femoral head and acetabulum. Two scenarios may be considered—persistent lateral hip subluxation and dislocation (Fig. 12). In the case of lateral hip subluxation, the pressure on the femoral head becomes concentrated along the medial aspect of the head as the hip hinges along the edge of the acetabulum. Likewise, concentric pressure on the acetabular floor is reduced while it is increased along the lateral edge. Since pressure inhibits appositional growth, the lateral femoral head continues to grow and flattens the head. The acetabular growth cartilage fills the acetabular floor and arrests its lateral growth, forming a progressively more shallow and oblique acetabulum. In the case of complete hip dislocation, both the head and acetabulum have unrestricted growth, yielding a large

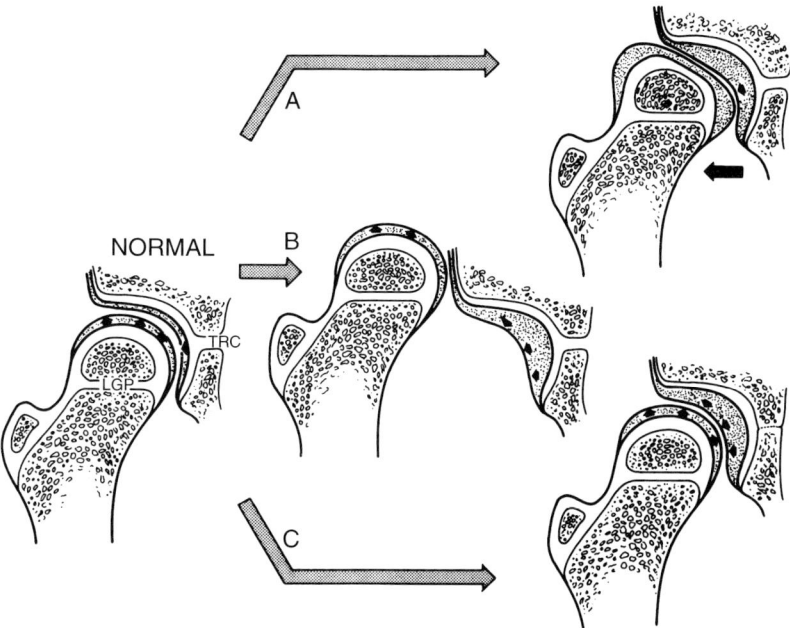

Fig. 12. The normal hip in child development is shown with the femoral head closely associated with the acetabulum to yield a congruent joint. When this relationship is lost, different acetabular deformities result. (*A*) depicts the deformity from lateral hip subluxation, (*B*) depicts the deformity from gross hip dislocation, and (*C*) depicts the deformity from early closure of the triradiate cartilage. (*Adapted from* Siffert RS. Patterns of deformity of the developing hip. Clin Orthop Relat Res 1981;Oct(160):20; with permission.)

head and a shallow acetabulum. With enough time, the femoral head no longer fits the socket and prevents reduction.

The treatment of DDH involves restoring the contact between femoral head and acetabulum. As the child ages, reduction of the dislocated or subluxated hip becomes increasingly difficult, often requiring closed or open procedures under general anesthesia. Restoration of normal acetabular development becomes less likely as the child ages; acetabular morphology is mostly determined by the age of 8 years [16,17].

Operative treatment of DDH often involves open reduction with pelvic and femoral osteotomies and offers another opportunity to apply principles of child hip development. Since the femoral head is typically large and the acetabulum is shallow in a subluxated or dislocated hip, it is thought that pelvic osteotomies that redirect rather than reshape the acetabulum are preferable. A reshaping osteotomy, such as the Pemberton, would decrease the already small acetabular volume and make difficult the maintenance of a reduction. Pelvic osteotomies may also disrupt the continued growth of the acetabulum (see Fig. 5). The operative procedure may cause closure of the triradiate cartilage. As a result, the medial wall of the acetabulum fails to grow and the acetabular articular cartilage cannot expand. A small, shallow acetabulum results, with a progressively subluxating femoral head.

In addition, varus femoral osteotomies for DDH offer an interesting study in proximal femoral growth dynamics. Loss of correction in varus osteotomy is commonly observed and is correlated to the age of the patient, with patients less than 4 years old showing the greatest loss in correction [26]. The remodeling of the varus proximal femur is related to the persistence of the growth plate and the dynamic reorientation of the physis with growth. Further, varus osteotomy may pose a risk to the greater trochanteric growth plate, leading to late deformity. Schofield and Smibert [27] reported an 18.8% reoperation rate for late valgus deformity in 11 of 14 patients in whom the greater trochanteric physis was violated during varus osteotomy.

Legg-Calvé-Perthes disease

Legg-Calvé-Perthes disease (LCPD) describes the apparently idiopathic progressive collapse and deformity of the femoral head in young children. LCPD is most common between the ages of 4 and 8 years, but may be seen in children as young as 2 years and as old as the early teens. It is more common in boys by a ratio of 4:1; and its international annual incidence is 1 in 1200 [24]. The etiology and late hip deformities of LCPD are particularly instructive on the growth and development of the child's hip.

The cause of LCPD is likely multifactorial, but most theories return to the tenuous vascular supply of the proximal femoral epiphysis. The peak incidence of LCPD between 4 to 8 years of age corresponds to specific anatomic vascular development peculiarities, as noted in the previous section from Chung's studies [20]. First, the epiphyseal and metaphyseal branches of the lateral ascending cervical artery, contributing the bulk of the blood supply to the proximal femoral epiphysis, originate from a single vessel that crosses the capsule at the trochanteric notch. Because the space between the trochanter and femoral neck is very narrow in children under eight years old, this single artery is vulnerable to occlusion by compression through hip positioning or unidentified exogenous sources [20]. Next, fewer arteries are present along the anterior and medial femoral neck in specimens from 3- to 10-year-old children than from newborn to 2-year-old children. Finally, the subsynovial intracapsular arterial supply is more often incomplete in males than in females, and may explain why LCPD is more common in boys. Blood supply to the epiphysis from the ligamentum teres likely does not impact the disease course of LCPD, because this supply is not related to age, sex, or race [20].

The pattern of venous drainage of the proximal femur has not been discussed in the vascular development of the proximal femur, but it has been implicated as a causative factor of LCPD. Heikkinen and colleagues noted abnormal venous patterns in 46 of 55 hips during the initial and fragmentation phases of LCPD [28]. Green and Griffin [29] demonstrated impaired patterns of venous outflow in 23 patients who had LCPD when compared with 23 normal hips. Liu and Ho [30] demonstrated delayed venous emptying from the femoral neck in 32 patients who had unilateral LCPD and reproduced lesions histologically similar to LCPD in skeletally immature dogs using an intraosseous injection of silicone into the femoral neck to impair venous outflow.

The altered growth of the femoral head in LCPD illustrates the deformity that may result with alterations in the longitudinal growth plate (LGP) and epiphyseal growth plate of the femoral head. Premature physeal plate closure occurs with LCPD and may be located either centrally or peripherally. In both cases, trochanteric overgrowth occurs. In central growth arrest, however, a short neck results without significant angular deformity. In lateral growth arrest, the femoral head and growth plate are tilted exter-

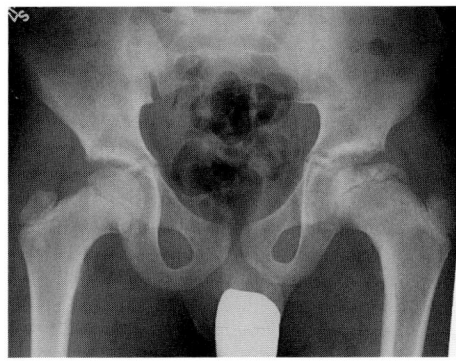

Fig. 13. Anteroposterior pelvic radiograph of a 9-year-old boy who has Legg-Calvé-Perthes disease, demonstrating the late deformity of a wide femoral neck, flattened and overgrown femoral head, and corresponding acetabular irregularity.

nally. Further, the deepest layer of articular cartilage ceases to grow, because it derives its nourishment from the epiphyseal blood vessels. The more superficial layer, which derives its nourishment from the synovial fluid, continues to grow and ossify, leading to a coxa magna. The FNI grows throughout the process and may yield a wide femoral neck (Fig. 13). With progressive deformity of the femoral head and neck, the femoral head is no longer containable; and motion is allowed only in the flexion and abduction plane. The lateral aspect of the acetabulum and the femoral head may be deformed secondarily by hinged abduction.

As in DDH, age and growth potential weigh heavily on the ability to restore a congruent joint. Young children with the disorder often demonstrate complete remodeling of the epiphysis. Even in cases of coxa magna, surgical containment procedures in this patient population can promote congruent development of the femur and acetabulum with respect to each other. On the other hand, children older than 8 years typically have a worse prognosis.

Summary

Child hip development is an ordered pathway of processes that results from the delicate interplay of cellular and mechanical influences. Critical to hip development is cell signaling, intrauterine differentiation and growth, and postnatal growth with maturation of its accompanying blood supply. Central to this process is the necessary contact between femoral head and acetabulum for congruent development. The sequelae of multiple disease processes and their treatments, including DDH and Legg-Calvé-Perthes disease, may be understood in the context of the growth history of this critical joint.

References

[1] Strayer Jr LM. Embryology of the human hip joint. Clin Orthop 1971;74:221–40.
[2] Watanabe RS. Embryology of the human hip. Clin Orthop 1974;98:8–26.
[3] Jouve JL, Glard Y, Garron E, et al. Anatomical study of the proximal femur in the fetus. J Pediatr Orthop B 2005;14(2):105–10.
[4] Fabry G, MacEwen GD, Shands AR. Torsion of the femur. J Bone Joint Surg Am 1973;55:1726–38.
[5] Zippel H. Untersuchungen zur normalentwicklung der formelemente am huftgelenk im wachstumsalter. [Normal development of the structural elements of the hip joint in adolescence]. Beitr Orthop 1971;18:255–70 [in German].
[6] Bobroff ED, Chambers HG, Sartoris DJ, et al. Femoral anteversion and neck-shaft angle in children with cerebral palsy. Clin Orthop Relat Res 1999;Jul(364):194–204.
[7] Macias D, Ganan Y, Sampath TK, et al. Role of BMP-2 and OP-1 (BMP-7) in programmed cell death and skeletogenesis during chick limb development. Development 1997;124(6):1109–17.
[8] Brunet LJ, McMahon JA, McMahon AP, et al. Noggin, cartilage morphogenesis, and joint formation in the mammalian skeleton. Science 1998;280(5368):1455–7.
[9] Storm EE, Kingsley DM. Joint patterning defects caused by single and double mutations in members of the bone morphogenetic protein (BMP) family. Development 1996;122(12):3969–79.
[10] Storm EE, Kingsley DM. GDF5 coordinates bone and joint formation during digit development. Dev Biol 1999;209(1):11–27.
[11] Thomas JT, Lin K, Nandedkar M, et al. A human chondrodysplasia due to a mutation in a TGF-beta superfamily member. Nat Genet 1996;12(3):315–7.
[12] Polinkovsky A, Robin NH, Thomas JT, et al. Mutations in CDMP1 cause autosomal dominant brachydactyly type C. Nat Genet 1997;17(1):18–9.
[13] Thomas JT, Kilpatrick MW, Lin K, et al. Disruption of human limb morphogenesis by a dominant negative mutation in CDMP1. Nat Genet 1997;17(1):58–64.
[14] Gilbert SF. Part 3. Later embryonic development. Chapter 16. Development of the tetrapod limb. In: Developmental biology. 6th edition. Sunderland (MA): Sinauer Associates, Inc.; 2000. p. 538–9.
[15] Ponseti IV. Growth and development of the acetabulum in the normal child. Anatomical, histological, and roentgenographic studies. J Bone Joint Surg Am 1978;60(5):575–85.

[16] Weinstein SL, Mubarak SJ, Wenger DR. Developmental hip dysplasia and dislocation. Part I. Instr Course Lect 2004;53:523–30.

[17] Weinstein SL, Mubarak SJ, Wenger DR. Developmental hip dysplasia and dislocation: Part II. Instr Course Lect 2004;53:531–42.

[18] Harrison TJ. The influence of the femoral head on pelvic growth and acetabular form in the rat. J Anat 1961;95:12–24.

[19] Siffert RS. Patterns of deformity of the developing hip. Clin Orthop Relat Res 1981;Oct(160):14–29.

[20] Chung SM. The arterial supply of the developing proximal end of the human femur. J Bone Joint Surg Am 1976;58(7):961–70.

[21] Crock HV. An atlas of the arterial supply of the head and neck of the femur in man. Clin Orthop Relat Res 1980;Oct(152):17–27.

[22] Parke WM. Chapter 1: the anatomy of the hip. In: Balderston RA, Rothman RH, Booth RE, et al, editors. The Hip. Philadelphia: Lea & Febige; 1992. p. 17–23.

[23] Lauritzen J. The arterial supply to the femoral head in children. Acta Orthop Scand 1974;45(5):724–36.

[24] Weinstein SL. Developmental hip dysplasia and dislocation. In: Buckwalter JA, Ehrlich MG, Sandell LJ, et al, editors. Skeletal growth and development: clinical issues and basic science advances. Rosemont (IL): American Academy of Orthopaedic Surgeons; 1998.

[25] Ponseti IV. Morphology of the acetabulum in congenital dislocation of the hip. Gross, histological and roentgenographic studies. J Bone Joint Surg Am 1978; 60(5):586–99.

[26] Brunner R, Baumann JU. Long-term effects of intertrochanteric varus-derotational osteotomy on femur and acetabulum in spastic cerebral palsy: an 11- to 18- year follow-up study. J Pediatr Orthop 1997;17(5): 585–91.

[27] Schofield CB, Smibert JG. Trochanteric growth disturbance after upper femoral osteotomy for congenital dislocation of the hip. J Bone Joint Surg Br 1990;72(1):32–6.

[28] Heikkinen E, Lanning P, Suramo I, et al. The venous drainage of the femoral neck as a prognostic sign in Perthes' disease. Acta Orthop Scand 1980;51(3):501–3.

[29] Green NE, Griffin PP. Intra-osseous venous pressure in Legg-Perthes disease. J Bone Joint Surg Am 1982; 64(5):666–71.

[30] Liu SL, Ho TC. The role of venous hypertension in the pathogenesis of Legg-Perthes disease. A clinical and experimental study. J Bone Joint Surg Am 1991;73(2): 194–200.

Evaluation of the Child Who Has Hip Pain

Steven L. Frick, MD

Carolinas Medical Center, P.O. Box 32861, Charlotte, NC 28232, USA

Children who have hip pathology can present in different ways, including complaints of pain, refusal to bear weight, limp or abnormal gait, or decreased movement of the lower extremity. The first thing to remember when considering lower extremity or gait complaints in skeletally immature patients is that patients who have hip pathology may present without complaining of hip pain. They may have a painless hip (developmental dysplasia of the hip, a shortened extremity) or complain of pain elsewhere (usually the knee or distal thigh). The pediatric population is challenging because some patients may be too young to complain of pain, and present with only decreased movement of the extremity or refusal to bear weight. Considering possible pathophysiologic categories during the evaluation can guide the clinician in the history taking, physical examination, and ordering of tests. The most common cause of lower extremity pain and limp in children is trauma; other categories to consider include inflammatory, infectious, developmental, and neoplastic processes (Table 1). Because developmental dysplasia of the hip does not usually present with pain in children, it is not covered here.

History

Obtaining a thorough history can be the most important part of the evaluation. Any recent traumatic events should be noted, and questions asked as to whether or not the child could ambulate after the trauma. Discovery of the onset, duration, severity, and location of the pain, and identifying factors that aggravate or alleviate the discomfort, can provide clues regarding etiology. Specific questioning should investigate associated systemic signs or symptoms, such as fever, sweating, and weight loss; and any recent infections or antibiotic usage should be recorded. To identify potentially serious causes of hip pain for which a timely diagnosis is essential, questions about night pain or rest pain should be asked. There are occasions in pediatric practice in which these questions are not answerable because of the patient's age, especially if the inciting event is not witnessed. In these cases, physical examination, imaging, and laboratory studies are needed to elucidate the diagnosis. The goal of targeted questions in the history is to assess the possibility that the pain is related to an infectious or neoplastic process, where delay in diagnosis and treatment can result in increased morbidity.

"Knee pain equals hip pain" is a maxim to consider in the patient who is skeletally immature, and important to remember in formulating a differential diagnosis and focusing the physical examination and possible imaging studies. This referred pain is thought to be a consequence of Hilton's Law—any nerve that passes over a joint sends some nerve fibers to innervate that joint. Thus the femoral nerve sends fibers to innervate the hip joint; and by way of referral pain pathways, hip pathology may present with the patient complaining of pain in the medial aspect of the thigh or knee, in the area of the terminal branch of the femoral nerve [1]. As an example, in one series up to 23% of patients who had slipped capital femoral epiphysis (SCFE) presented complaining only of knee pain [2]. Patients complaining of knee pain who are skeletally immature should be questioned specifically about associated hip or groin pain; and careful physical exam of the hips should be done, especially

E-mail address: steven.frick@carolinashealthcare.org

Table 1
Causes of lower extremity pain and limp in children

Traumatic/Mechanical	Infectious	Inflammatory	Vascular	Neoplastic
Fractures	Pyarthrosis	Transient synovitis	Legg-Calvé-Perthes disease	Benign aggressive tumors
Muscle injuries	Osteomyelitis	Juvenile rheumatoid arthritis	Osteonecrosis	Malignant tumors
Contusions	Pyomyositis	Ankylosing spondylitis	Hemoglobinopathies	Leukemia, lymphoma
SCFE Slipped capital femoral epiphysis	Lyme disease	Reiter syndrome		Benign tumors with impending fracture

when the knee examination is benign or nonfocal. Pelvic radiographs are obtained on patients complaining of knee pain if there is also any history of groin or hip pain, or an abnormality on hip examination.

Physical examination

Physical examination of the patient who has hip pain begins with recording vital signs, especially temperature. If able to ambulate, the child should be observed walking up and down a long hallway. Observational gait analysis should specifically look at the foot progression angle, at pelvic and trunk balance, and for presence or absence of a limp. The child who refuses to bear weight should be examined to see if sitting or crawling is tolerable. Inability to sit comfortably may point to spinal pathology, and ability to bear weight through the knees proximally when crawling can localize the problem to the legs or feet. Range of hip motion examination is critical, particularly looking for diminished or painful inward rotation. The anatomy of the hip joint is such that maximal intracapsular volume is possible with the hip in a position of flexion, abduction, and outward rotation. A febrile infant holding the hip in this position at rest likely needs an aspiration and arthrogram to rule out pyarthrosis. Conversely, the hip joint accommodates less intracapsular volume with extension, adduction, and inward rotation. If these passive motions cause pain, suspicion for an intra-articular process is heightened. Children who have irritable hips often allow a gentle "log-roll" inward and outward rotation of the extended lower extremity to assess side-to-side differences in hip rotation and guarding. A useful physical examination maneuver to rule out significant hip pathology is a supine active straight leg raise against resistance. The muscle contractions necessary to raise the lower extremity cause the hip joint to be loaded, and thus patients who can perform this movement easily, without pain and with symmetric strength, are unlikely to have hip joint pathology. Squatting to the ground and rising is a simple, fast test of active lower extremity joint motion and strength. Alternate single leg hopping can sometimes demonstrate subtle differences in side-to-side lower extremity function. Thigh atrophy (measured at a standard distance above the patella) can also be a subtle marker of long-standing hip pathology. If the patient's symptoms and physical examination signs are suspicious for hip pathology, laboratory studies and imaging may be indicated. Examination of other joints for swelling and skin examination for rashes can be helpful in identifying inflammatory or infectious causes of hip pain. Thorough palpation of the thigh is important to assess for any mass effect, and the inguinal area should be palpated also for any mass or lymphadenopathy.

Laboratory studies

Laboratory studies are used primarily for screening when the differential diagnosis includes infectious, inflammatory, or neoplastic processes. Most frequently ordered are a complete blood count (CBC) with differential, erythrocyte sedimentation rate (ESR), C-reactive protein (CRP), and rheumatoid panel (rheumatoid factor, ANA). A Lyme disease titer should be considered in endemic areas. Each test has literature discussing its use in evaluating limping children [3]. Some important caveats from that body of knowledge that are helpful in evaluating children who have hip pain are:

- The ESR and CRP are acute phase reactants, and either infectious, inflammatory, or neoplastic causes can result in elevation above normal levels. The CRP will increase and decrease faster than the ESR, and so may be a better marker of day-to-day progress when treating infections. Of note, the ESR and CRP are better negative predictors than positive predictors for infectious processes. One study of septic arthritis in

children found that patients who had a normal CRP had an 87% probability of not having septic arthritis [4].
- The rheumatoid panel may be normal, yet the patient may still have an inflammatory condition.
- Leukemia must be considered in the differential diagnosis in children who have musculoskeletal pain. Patients who have an elevated ESR and associated anemia, neutropenia, or thrombocytopenia may benefit from consultation with hematology/oncology colleagues and from bone marrow aspiration to diagnose leukemia [5].
- If an infectious etiology is suspected, a blood culture should be drawn at the time of other laboratory studies, because often the blood culture is the only positive culture in patients who have musculoskeletal infection. Patients do not have to be febrile at the time the blood culture is drawn.

Imaging

Anteroposterior radiography of the pelvis is the standard first-line imaging, preferably taken with the patient standing, if age and physical function allow. A centered, good-quality pelvic radiograph provides much information about the health and development of the hip joint and allows comparison of symptomatic and nonsymptomatic sides. Lateral views of both hips may be needed, depending on the differential diagnosis, because some conditions, such as early slipped capital femoral epiphysis or Legg-Calvé-Perthes disease (LCPD), may be more evident on the lateral view. Advanced imaging is helpful in cases in which infectious or neoplastic processes are suspected, and may include magnetic resonance imaging (MRI), computed tomography (CT) or nuclear medicine studies (bone scan, positive emission tomography scan). Nuclear imaging was described frequently in the 1990s as a method to elucidate the cause of nonspecific lower extremity pain and limping in children [6], but these methods require intravenous access, entail exposure to radiation, give nonspecific anatomic detail, and are not fast. MRI scanning has replaced nuclear imaging studies for the most part, because it can be done faster, does not expose the child to radiation, and can give greater anatomic detail [7]. Coronal screening images from the lumbar spine to the ankles can be obtained rapidly, looking for infectious or inflammatory processes in limping children. The disadvantage of MRI is that young children may require sedation or general anesthesia to acquire quality images. CT scans allow the images to be acquired much faster, but expose the child to radiation, making CT a less desirable choice for screening. CT is excellent if a bone abnormality is suspected, or if the area to be studied can be localized by physical exam or plain radiography. Ultrasound of the hip can be used to assess for a hip effusion, but it does not provide information differentiating inflammatory or traumatic effusions from infectious arthritis. Ultrasound also can be used to guide aspiration of the hip joint.

Traumatic and mechanical causes of hip pain

A history of trauma guides the physical examination and imaging studies to look for fractures, dislocations, muscle strains, or joint sprains. It is unusual for children to sprain or dislocate the hip joint, and fractures around the hip are caused typically by high-energy trauma and usually do not pose a diagnostic dilemma. An exception can be avulsion fractures of the pelvis, usually seen in older children and adolescents engaged in active sports. Focused examination reveals tenderness at sites of muscle attachment to the pelvis (anterior superior iliac spine – sartorius, anterior inferior iliac spine – rectus femoris, ischium – hamstrings) and pain on resisted strength testing of the involved muscles. Repetitive stress can also result in stress fractures of the femur that present with hip and thigh pain and may be confused with neoplastic processes such as Ewing's sarcoma. This confusion is because of the typical location (femoral diaphysis) and radiographic findings (periosteal reaction) that stress fractures in children and Ewing's sarcoma share. MRI can help distinguish between these two conditions, because stress fractures may have a visible disruption in cortical continuity and will not have an associated soft tissue mass or bone destruction, as is seen with sarcomas. Serial radiographic examinations reveal progressive healing of stress fractures after activity modification [8]. Repetitive motion of tendons over bone prominences can also cause symptoms, with snapping hip syndrome occurring from the psoas tendon abrading the pelvic brim and the tensor fascia lata/iliotibial band rubbing over the greater trochanter.

Slipped capital femoral epiphysis

SCFE is a disorder of the physis of the proximal femur, with the femoral neck slipping off the proximal femoral epiphysis, which is contained within the acetabulum. SCFE is more likely to occur in older children and adolescents and is felt to be primarily of mechanical etiology because it is typically seen in obese patients. It tends to occur between the ages of 10 and 16 years and is more common in boys. It is bilateral in approximately 20% of patients at the time of initial presentation, and another 20% to 30% will develop a contralateral slip within 12 to 18 months of the initial slip. As noted earlier, it often presents initially as knee pain, which can cause a delay in diagnosis. This delay can have significant consequences, because the degree of slip can increase during the delay, increasing the risk for arthritis and perhaps even of osteonecrosis, the most feared complication of SCFE. Patients who have SCFE are classified as having a stable or unstable slip, based on whether or not they can bear weight on the involved extremity [9]. The major difference prognostically between the two groups is the risk for osteonecrosis, which is negligible in patients who have stable SCFE, but increases to almost 50% in patients who have unstable SCFE. The goal of evaluation of ambulatory patients who have SCFE is to identify them and treat them (in situ screw stabilization) to prevent progression to an unstable SCFE with its concomitant increased risk for osteonecrosis, and to prevent further deformity of the proximal femur with its increased risk for developing osteoarthrosis. Patients who do not fit the typical profile of SCFE patients (younger age—less than 10 years—at presentation, body weight less than 50th percentile), should have an evaluation of renal and endocrine function, with hypothyroidism and growth hormone deficiency being the most common endocrinopathies associated with SCFE [10,11]. Patients who have SCFE usually have an asymmetrical outward foot progression angle on the involved side, have limited internal rotation, and may have obligatory outward rotation of the hip with flexion, to allow for clearance of the femoral neck, which would impinge on the anterior acetabulum with flexion in neutral rotation. The involved limb may be shortened. Radiographs confirm the diagnosis, with the lateral view being most sensitive for early slips of small magnitude. On the anteroposterior view, a line drawn along the superior femoral neck (Klein's line) should intersect some portion of the femoral head. Other subtle early signs are asymmetric physeal widening or blurring (blanch sign of Steel). In very suspicious cases by history and physical examination with normal initial radiographs, advanced imaging can be obtained (CT or MRI), or the patient can be placed on crutches with protected weight bearing and early return for repeat evaluation.

Inflammatory or infectious causes of hip pain

These two categories are presented together because the history and physical examination frequently leave these two as the leading possibilities, and clinical decision making in distinguishing between them is important, because the treatment needed is different.

When a child presents with an irritable hip, timely diagnosis is essential if the cause of the pain is septic arthritis of the hip [12]. An aphorism from Rang cautions the surgeon to "Never let the sun set on pus under pressure." Intra-articular infection can result in permanent loss of hip function, with early arthritis as a result of loss of articular cartilage, a shortened limb as a result of damage to growth cartilage, a hip dislocation as a result of distension and destruction of the joint capsule, or osteonecrosis and complete loss of the femoral head and neck as the worst-case scenario. The differentiation of septic arthritis from transient synovitis can be difficult, and no combination of tests has been found to be foolproof. As the sequelae of missed or late diagnosis can be severe, aggressive testing to rule out septic arthritis is favored, even though it is associated with some risks. Hip aspiration is regarded as the gold standard for diagnosis of septic arthritis, with positive findings on Gram stain and culture or the finding of greater than 50,000 white blood cells per mm^3 with a predominance of polymorphonuclear cells diagnostic. Because hip aspiration is painful, usually it is performed under sedation or general anesthesia; and it should be done under fluoroscopic guidance with arthrography or ultrasound confirmation to ensure that the hip joint is entered. A subadductor or anterior approach with a spinal needle can be used to enter the joint; and often in cases of septic arthritis, pus exits once the obturator is withdrawn. If synovial fluid is not encountered when the obturator is withdrawn and aspiration performed, the joint should be injected with radiographic contrast material to confirm intra-articular placement of the needle. Fluid that is withdrawn from the hip should be sent for cell count and differential, Gram stain, and culture. If no fluid is obtained on aspiration, the joint can be injected with a small amount (3–5 mL) of sterile saline, which is then reaspirated and sent for culture.

Because it is often not clear on presentation if infection is the cause of hip pain, the office evaluation of the child who has an irritable hip involves clinical decision making along the lines of threshold modeling described by Pauker and Kassirer [13]. The primary objective is to identify and treat all patients who have septic arthritis of the hip. The clinician has three options: (1) make a presumptive diagnosis of transient synovitis and order no further tests (observation threshold, treat with analgesics or anti-inflammatories), (2) order further testing (testing threshold) to elucidate the diagnosis (laboratory studies, imaging), or (3) proceed to invasive testing or treatment (test-treatment threshold) with hip aspiration/arthrogram or arthrotomy if suspicion for septic arthritis is high. Multiple studies have attempted to define factors that can be used to differentiate septic arthritis from transient synovitis of the hip. Noted factors include a history of fever, refusal to bear weight on the involved extremity, an elevated white blood cell (WBC) count in the peripheral blood, an elevated ESR, side-to-side differences in the width of the apparent hip joint space on radiographs, prior visits to a health care provider, and an elevated CRP [14–17]. Clinical decision rules based on these factors have a reported likelihood of identifying septic arthritis as high as 99% when a combination of these factors is used [14].

Transient synovitis of the hip is probably the most common cause of hip pain in children. Retrospective and prospective studies from large referral children's hospitals attempting to develop clinical algorithms to differentiate transient synovitis from septic arthritis have found patient populations that consist of two thirds with transient synovitis and one third with septic arthritis [14–16]. Patients who have septic arthritis tend to be younger on average; but there is a wide overlap, and septic arthritis of the hip can occur at any age. Transient synovitis typically occurs between the ages of 3 and 8 years, presenting with hip pain and a limp or even refusal to bear weight. It may be preceded by a viral illness or minor trauma, and it can have an acute or insidious onset. The child is usually not toxic in appearance, and typically does not have a high fever. Motion of the hip is usually possible in the midrange, with pain at the extremes. It is a benign, self-limited condition, with no known long-term sequelae. There are times, however, when patients present with fever, refusal to bear weight, and pain with any motion of the hip; and distinguishing transient synovitis from pyarthrosis is challenging.

Children who have septic arthritis of the hip usually appear ill, have a fever or a history of fever, refuse to bear weight, and guard against any movement of the involved hip. Transient bacteremic episodes are believed to result in deposition of bacteria within the hip joint and subsequent infection. Patients often have a history of mild antecedent trauma, which can be misleading; and some investigators have hypothesized that minor trauma may predispose the area to infection, as has been shown for osteomyelitis [18]. Again, the challenge is that patients who have septic arthritis may present early in the infectious process and not manifest the classic signs and symptoms.

Kocher and colleagues sought to provide a clinical decision-making algorithm based on a retrospective review of patients at Boston Children's Hospital over 17 years [14]. They identified four independent multivariate predictors of septic arthritis of the hip: a history of fever, inability to bear weight, an ESR of 40 mm/h or greater, and a serum WBC count greater than 12,000 cells/mm^3. Patient who had three of four predictors had a 93% chance of having septic arthritis, and those who had all four had a 99% likelihood of pyarthrosis.

Luhmann and colleagues [16] then looked at these four variables retrospectively in their patients from St. Louis Children's Hospital who underwent arthrocentesis for an irritable hip over an 8-year period and found that the presence of all four Kocher predictors in their patients predicted septic arthritis only 59% of the time. In their patients, statistical analysis revealed the three best predictors of septic arthritis were a history of fever, a serum WBC greater than 12,000 cells/mm^3, and a previous health care visit, with a probability of septic arthritis 71% of the time when all three variables were present. They questioned whether clinical decision algorithms developed in one center were valid if applied in a different health care setting. Jung and colleagues [17] performed a similar study to the retrospective study of Kocher and colleagues., and they identified five independent predictors of septic arthritis: a temperature of 37°C or greater, an ESR of 20 mm/h or greater, a CRP of greater than 1.0 mg/dL, a serum WBC of greater than 11,000/mm^3, and an apparent medial joint space difference of greater than or equal to 2mm on radiographs. Kocher and colleagues followed up their original study with a prospective study to validate their clinical prediction rule and found good diagnostic performance in these new patients. Patients who had zero of the four predictors had a 2% probability of septic arthritis, one of four 9.5%, two of four 35%, three of four 72.8%. Patients who had all four predictors present had a 93% probability of septic arthritis [15].

The clinical prediction rules of Kocher and colleagues are not meant to supplant clinical judgment, but they may be used to determine thresholds for clinical decision making as described by Kassirer and colleagues. Those patients who have three or four predictors may pass the test-treatment threshold and warrant hip aspiration/arthrogram. Experienced pediatric orthopedic surgeons believe there is no area more treacherous or more in need of a skilled and wise assessment than the evaluation of a child who has possible musculoskeletal infection about the hip.

Patients who have hip pain can have an infectious etiology and not have septic arthritis; the other sites of possible infection are the bones and muscles around the hip joint. Proximal femoral or pelvic osteomyelitis can present similarly to septic arthritis, although often the patients will still bear weight and allow some passive range of motion of the hip (less irritable). Osteomyelitis in either location around the joint can eventually erode into the joint and cause concomitant septic arthritis. This situation needs more timely diagnosis and treatment, because the effects of infection on articular cartilage can have more severe and irreversible effects than infections isolated to the bone. As noted previously, patients who have musculoskeletal infection may have had minor preceding trauma, which may predispose them to infection by providing an area of hematoma or injured tissue for bacteria to invade [18]. Pyomyositis, in particular, can mimic septic arthritis; and it should be kept in mind if hip aspiration or arthrogram is negative and the patient continues to manifest signs of infection (fever, positive blood cultures). Deep muscles around the pelvis can become infected (psoas, obturator internus, adductor brevis, gluteus minimus, and others) and present with pain around the groin, guarding against hip motion that stretches the involved muscle, and often fever or systemic illness. Typically ESR and CRP are elevated. MRI scanning is the best imaging study to assess for intramuscular abscesses, although CT scans can also be diagnostic [19,20].

Other infectious causes of hip pain include Lyme disease, although hip involvement is rare. It should be suspected in patients who have a history of a bull's-eye rash, a tick bite, or being in an area endemic for Lyme disease. Diagnosis is made by measurement of serum Lyme disease titer.

Inflammatory causes of childhood hip pain from juvenile rheumatoid arthritis, ankylosing spondylitis, or Reiter syndrome are uncommon. Family history of inflammatory or autoimmune conditions should be sought, and other joints should be examined for any signs of inflammation. Hip involvement in juvenile rheumatoid arthritis is uncommon except in the systemic form.

Reiter syndrome and ankylosing spondylitis rarely manifest in children and are more common in adolescents and young adults.

Vascular causes

LCPD is idiopathic osteonecrosis of the proximal femoral epiphysis. It is most commonly seen in children aged 4 to 8 years, and it occurs more often in boys. Some associations have been noted with delayed bone age, hyperactivity, and passive smoke inhalation. Some controversy exists regarding the presence of thrombophilia in patients who have LCPD, with conflicting studies published. It frequently presents initially with a painless limp, but then patients may develop pain, typically in concert with femoral head collapse. Patients may complain of pain in the hip, thigh, or knee. Patients often have pain at the end range of motion, especially abduction and internal rotation, with less painful midrange motion. Symptoms and limp severity are usually worse at the end of the day. The diagnosis of LCPD is made based on the radiographic appearance, with the earliest signs being a decreased size of one proximal femoral epiphysis, or increased density of one epiphysis. The lateral radiograph of the hip is more likely to show a crescent sign, a subchondral fracture that correlates with the extent of necrotic bone. Bilateral involvement is uncommon in patients who have LCPD; and when it is bilateral, there is usually sequential involvement. In patients who have symmetric flattening or fragmentation, multiple epiphyseal dysplasia or spondyloepiphyseal dysplasia should be considered. Prognosis for patients who have LCPD is most closely associated with age at presentation, and treatment generally follows containment principles [21].

Osteonecrosis of the proximal femoral epiphysis may also occur following fractures or dislocations of the hip, or after surgery around the hip. Other causes of osteonecrosis of the hip include hemoglobinopathies, such as sickle cell disease or thalassemia, leukemia, lymphoma, and hemophilia.

Neoplastic conditions

Several neoplastic conditions can present with hip pain. Most concerning of these are malignant neoplasms, particularly osteosarcoma and Ewing's sarcoma. Patients who have night or rest pain, systemic symptoms, or palpable masses should be evaluated with laboratory studies and imaging to assess for neoplasms. Benign neoplasms (bone cysts, fibrous dysplasia) that compromise the structural integrity of the bone may present with mechanical pain; and benign aggressive neoplasms, such as osteoid osteoma or chondroblastoma, may present with night pain and pain with weight bearing [22].

Leukemia is the most common malignancy in childhood and often presents with musculoskeletal complaints. One study noted the hip as the most frequent site of pain [5]. Thus, leukemia should be included in the differential diagnosis of limping children or patients who have hip pain, especially in patients who are initially believed to have an infectious etiology but do not improve during standard therapy for septic arthritis or osteomyelitis. Bone and joint pain is believed to be caused by the mass effect of malignant blast cells within the medullary canal. As malignant cells occupy the marrow space, the production of normal blood components is decreased and can offer diagnostic clues when assessing a patient who has hip pain on laboratory studies. Leukemic patients often have a very elevated ESR, with associated anemia, neutropenia, or thrombocytopenia. Often radiographs are normal, but MRI scans show the marrow replacement.

Summary

Evaluation of hip pain in children can be challenging, because there are several diagnoses to consider and differentiating among them can be difficult. Patients who have traumatic or mechanical causes of hip pain are not usually as difficult to diagnose, as long as the potential pitfall of referred pain to the knee is recognized, and appropriate radiographs are ordered and interpreted correctly. The diagnostic dilemma most commonly encountered involves identifying the etiology of the irritable hip in a child in whom the differential includes infectious, inflammatory, and neoplastic categories. A systematic approach based on the level of intensity of presenting circumstances can be helpful to guide the workup, allowing for clarification of the diagnosis without excessive use of testing that can be anxiety-provoking and costly and entails some risk to the patient. This approach is similar to the levels proposed by Wenger for evaluation of back pain in children [23]; and the predictors identified by Kocher and colleagues [14,15] are helpful, as long as it is recognized that they may not apply to every patient and may not be as predictive in settings outside Boston [16].

Patients who do not have systemic symptoms or signs and who on examination are considered to have a mild to moderately irritable hip may not pass the observation threshold. They are provisionally diagnosed as having transient synovitis and can be managed with analgesics and anti-inflammatory medications. Parents are given explicit instructions to return night or day for fever or increasing pain, and the patient is rechecked in 24 to 48 hours. Transient synovitis typically improves rapidly, and patients are often better within days. The course can be prolonged in a few patients, lasting up to three weeks. Those patients who do not improve rapidly may need more testing, particularly radiographs to look for subtle signs of LCPD disease. Patients who have two or more Kocher predictors, or a more irritable hip on examination, exceed the testing threshold; and laboratory studies and radiographs are obtained. Normal range findings on the ESR and CRP are supportive of a noninfectious etiology. Patients who have three or more Kocher predictors, systemic signs, or a severely irritable hip on examination pass the test-treatment threshold. Laboratory studies and radiographs are ordered, and clinical judgment determines whether the findings of all data gathered lead to advanced imaging (if the findings are not specific enough to the hip) or if the patient proceeds directly to aspiration-arthrogram and possible arthrotomy of the hip. Patients who have classic signs of septic arthritis who do proceed to arthrotomy and have either unimpressive findings at arthrotomy or negative cultures, should be evaluated with further imaging (pyomyositis, osteomyelitis) or even bone marrow aspiration (leukemia), if the patient does not improve on antibiotics.

References

[1] Wenger D. Knee pain in children and adolescents. In: Wenger D, Rang M, editors. The art and practice of children's orthopaedics. New York: Raven Press; 1993. p. 223.

[2] Matava J, Patton C, Luhmann S, et al. Knee pain as the initial symptom of slipped capital femoral epiphysis: an analysis of initial presentation and treatment. J Pediatr Orthop 1999;19:455–60.

[3] Flynn J, Widmann R. The limping child: evaluation and diagnosis. J Am Acad Orthop Surg 2001;9(2): 89–98.

[4] Levine M, McGuire K, McGowan K, et al. Assessment of the test characteristics of C-reactive protein for septic arthritis of the hip. J Pediatr Orthop 2003;23: 373–7.

[5] Tuten R, Gabos P, Kumar J, et al. The limping child:

[5] a manifestation of acute leukemia. J Pediatr Orthop 1998;18(5):625–9.
[6] Aronson J, Garvin K, Seibert J, et al. Efficiency of bone scan for occult limping toddlers. J Pediatr Orthop 1992;12:38–44.
[7] White P, Boyd J, Beattie T, et al. Magnetic resonance imaging as the primary imaging modality in children presenting with acute non-traumatic hip pain. Emerg Med J 2001;18(1):25–9.
[8] Lee S, Baek J, Han S, et al. Stress fracture of the femoral diaphysis in children: a report of 5 cases and review of the literature. J Pediatr Orthop 2005;25(6):734–8.
[9] Loder R, Richards B, Shapiro P, et al. Acute slipped capital femoral epiphysis: the importance of physeal stability. J Bone Joint Surg Am 1993;75:1134–40.
[10] Loder R, Wittenberg B, DeSilva G. Slipped capital femoral epiphysis associated with endocrine disorders. J Pediatr Orthop 1995;15:349–56.
[11] Loder R, Greenfield M. Clinical characteristics of children with atypical and idiopathic slipped capital femoral epiphysis: description of the age-weight test and implications for further diagnostic evaluation. J Pediatr Orthop 2001;21:481–7.
[12] Rang M. Infections and tumors. In: Wenger D, Rang M, editors. The art and practice of children's orthopaedics. New York: Raven Press; 1993. p. 598.
[13] Pauker S, Kassirer J. The threshold approach to clinical decision making. N Engl J Med 1980;302:1109–17.
[14] Kocher M, Zurakowski D, Kasser J. Differentiating between septic arthritis and transient synovitis of the hip in children. An evidence-based clinical prediction algorithm. J Bone Joint Surg Am 1999;81:1662–70.
[15] Kocher M, Mandiga R, Zurakowski D, et al. Validation of a clinical prediction rule for differentiation between septic arthritis and transient synovitis of the hip in children. J Bone Joint Surg Am 2004;86:1629–35.
[16] Luhmann S, Jones A, Schootman M, et al. Differentiation between septic arthritis and transient synovitis of the hip in children with clinical prediction algorithms. J Bone Joint Surg Am 2004;86:956–62.
[17] Jung S, Rowe S, Moon E, et al. Significance of laboratory and radiologic findings for differentiating between septic arthritis and transient synovitis of the hip. J Pediatr Orthop 2003;23(3):368–72.
[18] Morrissy R, Haynes DW. Acute hematogenous osteomyelitis: a model with trauma as an etiology. J Pediatr Orthop 1989;9:447–56.
[19] Hosalkar H, Chatoo M, Jones S, et al. Hip pain in a 6 year old girl. Clin Orthop 2004;419:311–5.
[20] Wong-Chung J, Bagali M, Kaneker S. Physical signs in pyomyositis presenting as a painful hip in children: a case report and review of the literature. J Pediatr Orthop B 2004;13:211–3.
[21] Herring J. Legg-Calvé-Perthes Disease. Rosemont (IL): American Academy of Orthopaedic Surgeons; 1996. p. 14–6 [monograph].
[22] Gebhardt M, Rosenthal D, Arnell P. Case 8–2005: A 10-year old boy with pain in the right thigh. N Engl J Med 2005;352:1122–9.
[23] Wenger D. Back pain in children and adolescents. In: Wenger D, Rang M, editors. The art and practice of children's orthopaedics. New York: Raven Press; 1993. p. 456–7.

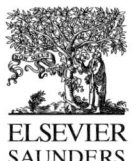

Role of Ultrasound in the Diagnosis and Management of Developmental Dysplasia of the Hip: An International Perspective

Marek Synder, MD, PhD[a,b,]*, H. Theodore Harcke, MD[c,d,e], Marcin Domzalski, MD[a]

[a]*Clinic of Orthopaedics and Pediatric Orthopaedics, Medical University of Lodz, Drewnowska Street 75, PL-91-002 Lodz, Poland*
[b]*Orthopaedic Department, Medical University of Lodz, Kosciuszki Street 4, 90-419 Lodz, Poland*
[c]*Department of Radiology, Jefferson Medical College, 1020 Walnut Street, Philadelphia, PA 19107-5587, USA*
[d]*Department of Pediatrics, Jefferson Medical College, 1020 Walnut Street, Philadelphia, PA 19107-5587, USA*
[e]*Alfred I. duPont Hospital for Children, 1600 Rockland Road, Wilmington, DE 19803, USA*

Late-diagnosed developmental dysplasia of the hip (DDH) has implications not only for the child and the family but also for the health care system [1,2]. Late-diagnosed DDH is particularly relevant in a geographic region where the population has a high prevalence of DDH [1,3]. Almost 10% of all total hip replacements are performed because of hip disorders of childhood, mostly DDH [2]. In countries that have developed a national program to diagnose DDH early, prevalences of late diagnosis and surgeries have been reduced [4–7]. A key element in those programs has been the use of ultrasound. In Poland, the prevalence of DDH is high (68 per 1000 births), and before 1985 there was a large number of late-diagnosed cases [3].

Early diagnosis of DDH is very important for proper and relatively easy treatment. Ultrasound has made this possible. Hip sonography allows one not only to visualize the cartilaginous parts of the newborn joints but also to observe the hip during motion [8–10]. This type of imaging of the neonatal hip has changed the understanding of and approach to DDH [11].

During the past 25 years, a variety of ultrasound techniques have been used for early diagnosis of DDH, but two of them are the most popular and widely used in the orthopedic practice: Graf's technique in Europe and Harcke's method in the United States [7–13]. In Poland, the authors instituted a combined clinical and ultrasound screening program in 1983 and have examined more than 60,000 infants. They incorporated the best practices of those who reported successful use of ultrasound in diagnosis and management of DDH [2,12,14].

Graf [10] was the first to introduce hip ultrasound to orthopedic practice. His method is based on the acetabular morphology of the hip joint and classification of the hip according to rigid guidelines of angular measurement (alpha and beta angles) [12].

Harcke's method, called "dynamic examination," is based on viewing the hip in multiple projections, including while the hip is in motion and being stressed [7–9]. Graf and Harcke agreed in 1993 on a merger of both methods and proposed a standard examination of the infant hip [15]. The principles of this basic examination mandate that the hip should be examined in the coronal plane at rest and in the transverse plane during the stress maneuvers. Both

---

This work was supported by Grant No. 503-115-1 from the Medical University of Lodz, Lodz, Poland.
* Corresponding author. Clinic of Orthopaedics and Pediatric Orthopaedics, Medical University of Lodz, Drewnowska Street 75, PL-91-002 Lodz, Poland.
E-mail address: msynder@pro.onet.pl (M. Synder).

the stability and the morphology of the hip joint should be evaluated; use of measurements remains optional. This standard enables assessment of hip position, morphology, and stability. In Poland, the dynamic examination of the newborn hip is used with the addition of measurements of alpha and beta angles [13].

This article reviews the role of ultrasound in diagnosis and management of DDH with an emphasis on its practice in Poland, where there is a high prevalence of hip dysplasia. Described is an approach to diagnosis and treatment of DDH, compared with international methods. Poland was the first East European country to institute a national program using ultrasound for newborn hip examination. The program drew on the experience of researchers in Europe and the United States.

Advantages of hip ultrasonography

The ultrasonographic examination has many advantages. It is safe, inexpensive, and easy to perform and does not involve ionizing radiation. Ultrasound equipment was initially available in Poland only in large hospitals and some clinics. Availability continued to increase, and in 1994 all health facilities had ultrasound equipment. The ultrasound examination enables one to distinguish the cartilaginous elements of the hip joint from the other soft tissue structures surrounding the joint. Ultrasonography affords the possibility to see the hip joint during movement and in multiplanar views.

Ultrasonography offers a number of advantages over the previously used radiologic methods. Because plain radiography of the pelvis is insufficient to visualize the immature hip during the first months of life, ultrasonography is able to fill the imaging gap in the diagnosis of DDH. Ultrasonography can be performed at an earlier age than radiography, whereas reliable radiographic changes require waiting until the infant is 3 to 4 months of age.

Ultrasonography is more sensitive than the clinical examination, even with an experienced orthopedic surgeon. Ultrasonography allows a physician to verify clinical findings, particularly in doubtful cases.

Screening of the hip joints

Presently, the main interest in the field of DDH is directed to the complex issue of screening. Orthopedic surgeons and pediatricians agree some type of screening is prudent, and the questions are as follows: what kind of screening, and when should it be done? Should one screen only by clinical examination and do selected cases with ultrasonography (eg, evidence of risk factors or abnormal physical examination), or should one screen all babies by ultrasonography independent of clinical findings?

Clinical screening for DDH was introduced in the 1960s, and this program is widely used in many countries [1,4,12–14,16–18]. The program consists of clinical examination of newborns by pediatricians or orthopedic surgeons in the hospital. Poland began routine clinical examination of all newborns in the 1970s [3], by orthopedic surgeons.

The initial optimism that clinical examination performed early would eliminate late-presenting cases of DDH was confronted by many studies [19,20]. Godward and Dezateux [21] found that 70% of children requiring surgery for hip dislocation had not been identified by clinical examination. Rosenberg and coworkers [22] and Rosenberg and Bialik [23], who found that clinical examination had failed to identify 63% of dislocated hips, presented similar findings.

The explanation of why clinical examination is inefficient is complex. DDH comprises a wide variety of abnormalities. Some hips present with only joint laxity, whereas others show only primary changes in the acetabulum. Ortolani and Barlow maneuvers are of great diagnostic value to detect dysplastic hips with joint laxity in newborns. From the authors' practice, however, it is known that these early symptoms of hip dysplasia disappear within the first few weeks of life. The only permanent DDH symptom may be limited abduction of the involved hip. The other findings of hip clicks and asymmetry of inguinal folds have been, for many years, the matter of controversy. Although most studies presented hip clicks as benign and without pathologic significance, some authors believed that clicks in a newborn are not always benign and should be closely monitored.

The authors' experience is the same as Nimityongskul and coworkers [5], who found an absence of abnormality using ultrasonography to examine newborns with clicks. The authors also believe that hip clicks are common during the first weeks of life. In their experience, asymmetry of the inguinal skin folds is frequently detected in newborns, but dysplasia of the hip was diagnosed in only 6% of children with this finding [24]. Some recommendations, however, suggest using this finding as a risk factor for screening purposes.

Some authors have described cases of DDH without any clinical symptoms [2,17,25]. This phenomenon, called "silent dysplasia," was widely discussed in the Polish orthopedic literature [2]. The typical prevalence of hip dysplasia without clinical symptoms is estimated to be 7% to 9%, but it has been reported to be as high as 22% [26]. Clinical screening alone has been ineffective in the detection of all cases of hip dysplasia [20,25]. This failure may reflect either inexperienced examiners or limitation in the clinical screening method [27,28]. These concerns about the reliability of clinical screening have resulted in the consideration of other methods to diagnose hip dysplasia [21]. Clinical examination as the only method of screening can be sufficient when performed by an experienced and appropriately trained examiner, but cases of primary acetabular dysplasia are still likely to be missed [27–29].

To improve the accuracy of clinical screening, certain risk factors of hip dysplasia, such as breech position, female gender, white race, family history, and postural deformities, have been described in the literature. In the 1980s, ultrasonography was added to the orthopedic diagnostic procedures, but indication for its use in newborn hip screening was not agreed on universally.

There are two primary approaches to DDH screening. First, universal infant screening was introduced in German-speaking countries (Germany, Austria, Switzerland) and central European countries (Poland and Czech Republic). The focus was on a newborn hip examination using the method described by Graf [10,12]. This examination produced a very high rate of positive studies and led to treatment rates beyond what was considered appropriate [2,9,16,17,30]. In one study from Norway, there was a large increase in the number who received treatment [31]. Graf's coronal view, equivalent to an anteroposterior radiograph of the hip, is the basis of his technique. Measurements of acetabular configuration (alpha and beta angles) are prescribed. The coronal view of the hip proposed by Graf is not difficult to find; however, reproducibility and reliability of both angles are controversial.

As a result of some reports in the literature, some programs for ultrasound screening were changed for children age 4 weeks or older. There is variability between countries on the exact timing of screening when it is delayed beyond the newborn period. In European countries, the continued focus on screening all infants is based on prevalence of DDH and the low cost of ultrasonographic studies. Synder and coworkers [2] and Synder and Zwierzchowski [13] in Poland proposed the use of the Graf and Harcke methods as one combined technique for hip examination. The authors believe Poland is the only country to use this combined technique.

A second screening plan established in the United States and England is based on newborn clinical examination with ultrasound examination used as a diagnostic tool in selected cases. Studies of selective screening showed that not all cases are detected. Boeree and Clarke [4] reported late cases at a rate of 1 per 5000.

The United States has rejected universal screening because of the cost versus benefit in a large, diverse population without a unified health care system [32]. Guidelines indicate repeated clinical examination with ultrasonography as an adjunct to the clinical evaluation at the discretion of the examiners [33].

Before a screening program was introduced to the orthopedic practice, the rate of surgery for late-diagnosed dislocation of the hip joint ranged from 1.6 to 2.1 per 1000 infants [2,4,26]. With the use of ultrasound, the rate has been reduced to 0.2 per 1000 [2,4,16]. Lewis and coworkers [34] also reported a marked decrease in the number of late-diagnosed DDH from 2.2 in 1000 to 0.34 in 1000 births using only the selective ultrasound screening, which included 15% of the population with risk factors. This also reduced the total cost of treatment of the children with DDH. Clegg and coworkers [18] demonstrated a decrease in costs from £5110 to £468 per 1000 births after ultrasonography was used for diagnostic procedures.

Based on the clinical experience in Poland, the authors adopted a program for screening all infants with the standard hip examination and using ultrasonography. First, all newborns are examined clinically at the hospital by the orthopedic surgeon or pediatrician at the age of 2 to 3 days for hip stability and physical clues of dysplasia. Babies with an abnormal hip examination have ultrasonography performed and are scheduled for observation, follow-up hip ultrasonography, or treatment. The authors identified 6 weeks of age as the optimal timing for the first ultrasonographic examination of all infants with a normal newborn clinical examination. In the authors' opinion, earlier screening could lead to a high false-positive rate of dysplasia because, at that age, a number of infants are found with only minor abnormality of the hip joint. This abnormality, instability, or acetabular dysplasia resolved at a later age. Marks and coworkers [35] performed initial ultrasound scanning at 48 hours of life and saw a 90% normalization of abnormal scans by the age of 4 to 6 weeks. The authors also recommend performing the ultrasonographic hip screening at the age of 6 weeks to prevent unidentified cases of hip dysplasia that remain undetected because the dysplasia developed after the newborn period. At the age of 6 weeks, there

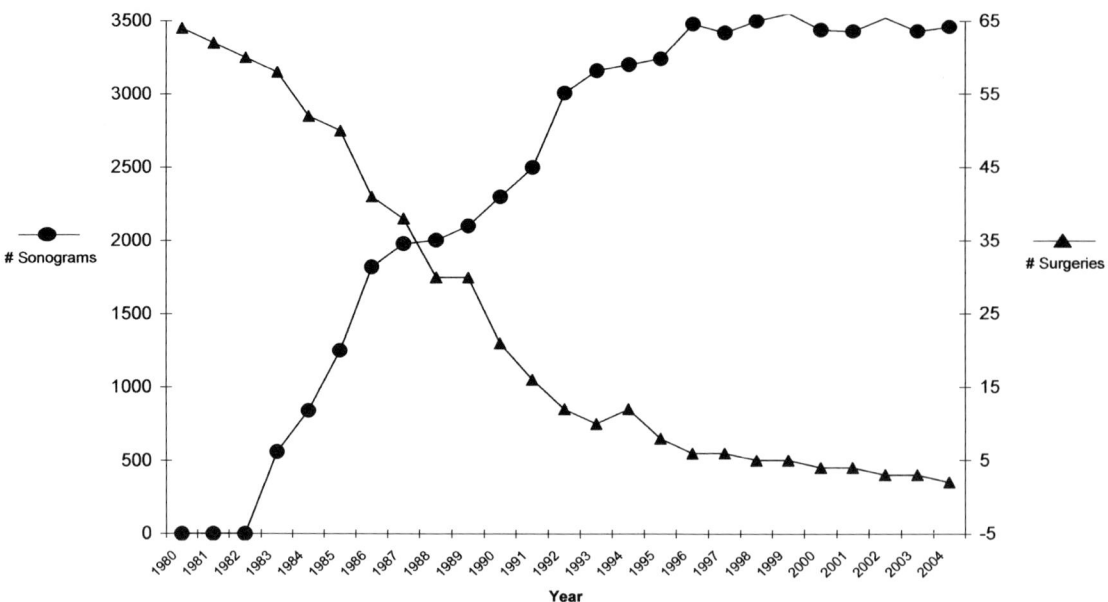

Fig. 1. Diagram showing the decreasing number of hip operations after the ultrasonographic techniques were introduced in the Clinic of Pediatric Orthopaedics, Medical University of Lodz, Poland.

is still enough time to begin treatment and have a good outcome.

When early screening leads to unnecessary treatment, it is important to modify protocols by either repeating the examination in 2 to 4 weeks or by delaying the ultrasound. Avoidance of abduction splinting is important, because it has recognized side effects, including avascular necrosis of the femoral head, tibial torsion, and femoral nerve palsy [2,21,22].

Experience in Poland supports general screening of the hip joints at age 6 weeks with clinical and ultrasound examination as a follow-up to the newborn clinical examination (Fig. 1). It is a successful plan because it initially captures all babies, it is cost-effective, and it does not result in overtreatment. Other countries with high rates of DDH and a health care system similar to Poland's should find this protocol effective.

Who should perform the ultrasound examination?

One of the most important questions concerning hip sonography is who should perform the ultrasound examination. The proper use of this tool requires training and experience. In different countries, orthopedic surgeons, pediatricians, radiologists, and general practitioners perform the ultrasonography.

In Europe, usually orthopedic surgeons or pediatricians perform sonography of the hip joint, whereas in the United States radiologists usually do this examination. In Poland, hip sonography is performed mainly by orthopedic surgeons. This approach to the ultrasound examination allows the orthopedic surgeon good correlation with clinical examination and an ability to monitor treatment directly. All orthopedic residents in Poland are taught to do hip sonography while in training, under the supervision of a qualified attending. Pediatricians and pediatric surgeons are instructed on DDH and when to refer infants for consultation.

Management of developmental dysplasia of the hip using ultrasound

Treatment options for DDH are very similar in many countries. In Poland, clinicians start with a clinical examination of the neonatal hips during the first 2 to 3 days of life to check for stability and clinical signs of dysplasia. Babies with normal hips at clinical examination are scheduled for ultrasound screening at the age of 6 weeks. All babies with abnormal hips on newborn clinical examination are placed under orthopedic observation, and selected cases are sent for ultrasound examination and treatment.

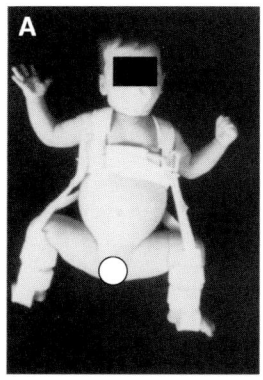
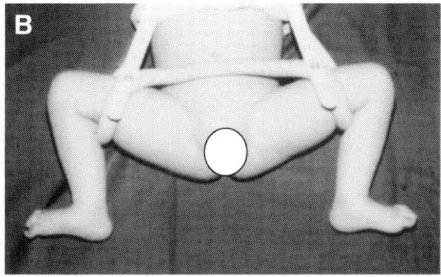

Fig. 2. Devices most commonly used in Poland for initial treatment of developmental dysplasia of the hip. (*A*) Pavlik harness. (*B*) Koszla splint.

Hips with evidence of dysplasia without displacement are treated initially with triple diapers. In the treatment protocol, the authors use triple diapers in infants with laxity (Barlow test positive, but Ortolani negative) for 3 to 6 weeks. Resistant instability during the next 2 to 3 weeks with diaper treatment is an indication to change the treatment and put an infant in Pavlik harness, which is worn until the hip is stable and the sonogram shows normalization of the hip joint.

The authors usually recommend having a child wear the harness for an additional 2 weeks after the hip becomes stable. Subluxated or dislocated hips are immediately treated with the Pavlik harness or other abduction devices, starting with a full-time regimen for the first 4 to 6 weeks (Fig. 2). Every second week, the child is examined clinically for hip stability and by ultrasound to monitor hip stability and acetabular remodeling (angle measurements). The monitoring of the hips is performed until the dysplastic hip is normal [36]. When the Pavlik harness is used, progress is expected to be seen in 2 to 3 weeks. If ultrasound shows no progress, the infant undergoes traction and closed or open reduction.

From the authors' experience, one can generalize the average time required for hip remodeling according to the Graf classification. In type IIA, the average time for hip remodeling is 3 weeks, and for type IIB it is 5 weeks. More severe types of hip dysplasia require a longer period of time for the full remodeling of the hip. In type IID, 8 weeks is required for hip rebuilding, and for types IIIa and IIIb, 14 and 18 weeks are required, respectively. The time necessary to rebuild the dislocated hips (type IV according to Graf classification system) averages 24 weeks (Fig. 3). The authors have found that 5% of all hips classified as types IIIb and IV do not respond to treatment (Pavlik harness, overhead traction, and so forth) and are scheduled for an operation. Radiographs are used after age 1 year, and all children are observed periodically after treatment until age 18 years.

The authors' observations are similar to those presented by Hangen and coworkers [37]. They found

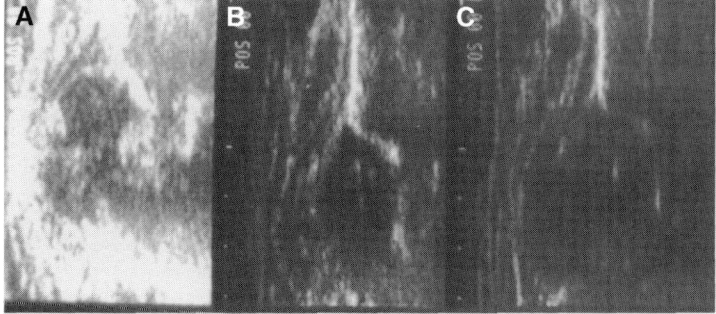

Fig. 3. Monitoring of the displaced hip of a newborn first seen at the age of 6 weeks. (*A*) Sonogram at the age of 6 weeks. (*B*) Two months later with the treatment with Pavlik harness (hip stable but with severe dysplastic signs of acetabulum). (*C*) Full remodeling of the hip joint at the age of 6 months.

a significantly shorter treatment time in infants with hip dysplasia who were followed by ultrasound monitoring than in those who did not have ultrasound examination [37].

Summary

The use of ultrasound for diagnosis and management of infant hip dysplasia has gained wide acceptance internationally. Poland has instituted a DDH screening program that incorporates ultrasound with two clinical examinations. The orthopedic surgeon conducts clinical examinations and sonograms, a practice that differs from many countries. The first clinical examination is performed at birth, and ultrasound and a second clinical examination are done at age 6 weeks. Experience since 1983 has led the authors to use an ultrasound technique that combines the methods of Harcke and Graf.

Treatment protocol indicates use of triple diapers (3–6 weeks) for infants with laxity. Pavlik harness is used with displaced hips and acetabular dysplasia. Unsuccessful Pavlik treatment is followed with overhead traction and closed or open reduction. Ultrasound has reduced the number of late-presenting cases, shortened treatment time, and decreased the number of surgical procedures of the hip joint in Poland.

References

[1] Bialik V, Bialik GM, Blazer S, et al. Developmental dysplasia of the hip: a new approach to incidence. Pediatrics 1999;103:93–9.
[2] Synder M, Niedzielski K, Grzegorzewski A. Ultrasonography of the newborn and infant hip. Ortopedia Tarumatologia Rehabilitacja 2003;6:117–21.
[3] Szulc W. The frequency of occurance of congenital dysplasia of the hip in Poland. Clin Orthop 1991;272: 100–2.
[4] Boeree NR, Clarke NM. Ultrasound imaging and secondary screening for congenital dislocation of the hip. J Bone Joint Surg Br 1994;76:525–33.
[5] Nimityongskul P, Hudgens RA, Anderson LD, et al. Ultrasonography in the management of developmental dysplasia of the hip. J Pediatr Orthop 1995; 15:741–6.
[6] Roovers EA, Boere-Boonekamp MM, Castelein RM, et al. Effectiveness of ultrasound screening for developmental dysplasia of the hip. Arch Dis Child Fetal Neonatal Ed 2005;90:25–30.
[7] Harcke HT, Kumar SJ. The role of ultrasound in the diagnosis and management of congenital dislocation and dysplasia of the hip. J Bone Joint Surg Am 1991; 73:622–8.
[8] Harcke HT. Screeing newborns for developmental dysplasia of the hip: the role of sonography. AJR Am J Roentgenol 1994;162:395–7.
[9] Harcke HT. Imaging methods used for children with hip dysplasia. Clin Orthop 2005;434:71–7.
[10] Graf R. The diagnosis of congenital hip-joint dislocation by the ultrasonic Combound treatment. Arch Orthop Trauma Surg 1980;97:117–33.
[11] Roposch A. Twenty years of hip ultrasonography: are we doing better today? J Pediatr Orthop 2003;23: 691–2.
[12] Graf R. Classification of hip joint dysplasia by means of sonography. Arch Orthop Trauma Surg 1984;102: 248–55.
[13] Synder M, Zwierzchowski TJ. Ultrasound diagnosis of the neonatal hips using the Harcke's method in newborns and infants. Chir Narzadow Ruchu Ortop Pol 1995;60:281–5.
[14] Zwierzchowski TJ, Zwierzchowski H, Synder M. The reliability of Graf's and Harcke's techniques in the prophylaxis of DDH. Chir Narzadow Ruchu Ortop Pol 1996;61(Suppl 3A):145–50.
[15] Harcke HT, Grissom LE. Infant hip sonography: current concepts. Semin Ultrasound CT MR 1994;15: 256–63.
[16] Vane AG, Jones DP, Dunbar JD, et al. The diagnosis and management of neonatal hip instability: results of a clinical and targeted ultrasound screening program. J Pediatr Orthop 2005;25:292–5.
[17] Lowry CA, Donoghue VB, Murphy JF. Auditing hip ultrasound screening of infants at increased risk of developmental dysplasia of the hip. Arch Dis Child 2005;90:579–81.
[18] Clegg J, Bache CE, Raut VV. Financial justification for routine ultrasound screening of the neonatal hip. J Bone Joint Surg Br 1999;81:852–7.
[19] Barlow TG. Early diagnosis and treatment of congenital dislocation of the hip. J Bone Joint Surg Br 1982; 44:291–301.
[20] Sanfridson J, Redlund-Johnell I, Uden A. Why is congenital dislocation of the hip still missed? Analysis of 96,891 infants screened in Malmo 1956–1987. Acta Orthop Scand 1991;62:87–91.
[21] Godward S, Dezateux C. Surgery for congenital dislocation of the hip in the UK as a measure of outcome of screening. Lancet 1998;351:1149–52.
[22] Rosenberg N, Bialik V, Norman D, et al. The importance of combined clinical and sonographic examination of instability of the newborn hip. Int Orthop 1998;22:185–8.
[23] Rosenberg N, Bialik V. The effectiveness of combined clinical-sonographic screening in the treatment of neonatal hip instability. Eur J Ultrasound 2002;15:55–60.
[24] Zwierzchowski H, Garncarek P, Synder M. Die beurteilung der positiven huftdysplasiezeichen im vergleich mit ultrasonographischenn bildern bei sauglingen. Orthop Praxis 1988;12:736–8.

[25] Jones D. An assessment of the value of examination of the hip in newborn. J Bone Joint Surg Br 1997;59: 318–22.
[26] Czeizel E, Vizkelety T. Incidence of congenital hip dislocation in Hungary. Orv Hetil 1988;129:2605–7.
[27] Macnicol MF. Results of a 25-year screening program for neonatal hip instability. J Bone Joint Surg Br 1990;72:1057–60.
[28] Poul J, Bajerova J, Summernitz M, et al. Early diagnosis of congenital dislocation of the hip. J Bone Joint Surg Br 1992;74:695–700.
[29] Darmonov AV, Zagora S. Clinical screening for congenital dislocation of the hip. J Bone Joint Surg Am 1996;78:383–7.
[30] Paton RW, Srinivasan MS, Shah B, et al. Ultrasound screening for hips at risk in developmental dysplasia of the hip: is it worth it? J Bone Joint Surg Br 1999; 81:225–8.
[31] Hinderaker T, Daltveit AK, Irgens LM, et al. The impact of intrauterine factors on neonatal hip instability: an analysis of 1,059,479 children in Norway. Acta Orthop Scand 1994;65:239–42.
[32] Lehmann HP, Hinton R, Morello P, et al. Developmental dysplasia of the hip practice guidelines: technical report. Pediatrics 2000;105:E57–63.
[33] American Academy of Pediatrics. Clinical practice guideline: early detection of developmental dysplasia of the hip. Pediatrics 2000;105:896–905.
[34] Lewis K, Jones DA, Powell N. Ultrasound and neonatal hip screening: the five-year results of prospective study in high-risk babies. J Pediatr Orthop 1999;19: 760–2.
[35] Marks DS, Clegg J, al-Chalabi AN. Routine ultrasound screening for neonatal hip instability: can it abolish late-presenting congenital dislocation of the hip? J Bone Joint Surg 1994;76:534–8.
[36] Niedzielski K, Synder M, Bira M. Monitoring of the rebuilding of the dysplastic hips with the use of ultrasound. Biblioteka Ortopedii Dziecięcej Tom VIII, Lublin 2002;8:9–15.
[37] Hangen DH, Kasser JR, Emans JB, et al. The Pavlik harness and developmental dysplasia of the hip: has ultrasound changed treatment patterns? J Pediatr Orthop 1995;15:729–35.

Treatment of Developmental Dysplasia of the Hip After Walking Age With Open Reduction, Femoral Shortening, and Acetabular Osteotomy

Edilson Forlin, MD, MSc, PhD[a,b],*, Luiz A. Munhoz da Cunha, MD, MSc, PhD[a,b], Daniel C. Figueiredo, MD[a]

[a]Hospital Pequeno Principe, Rua Desembargador Motta, 1070, CEP 80250-060, Curitiba, PR, Brazil
[b]Hospital das Clinicas da UFPR, Rua General Carneiro, 181 Centro, CEP 80060-900, Curitiba, PR, Brazil

Untreated developmental dysplasia of the hip (DDH) in the older child has become uncommon in the first world, but it is still seen in developing countries. The goals of operative treatment in older children do not differ from those in young patients: to obtain a well-reduced and stable hip; to correct acetabular dysplasia, and to avoid complications, such as avascular necrosis. With these goals assured, physicians can then provide optimal conditions for appropriate development of the joint and, consequently, an excellent functional performance in the long term.

The abnormalities of a dislocated hip become more pronounced with age. Anterior acetabular deficiency is still preponderant; however, posterior or global deficiencies are also common. The transverse acetabular ligament hypertrophies, narrowing the acetabulum entrance. Under the stress of weight-bearing, the capsule hypertrophies and becomes an important obstacle. It may also adhere to the outer wall of the ilium. The femoral head can be flat posteromedially and become deformed. Increased femoral anteversion is present in varying degrees. The acetabulum becomes progressively thick, shallow, and oblique with excessive antetorsion. With time and progression of the displacement, the muscles and soft tissues around the hip become shortened and contracted. The psoas tendon may also constrict the capsule. As the deformity progresses, operative correction becomes more difficult, and the rates of poor results and complications increase.

There is much controversy regarding treatment in children older than the age of two years. Traction before the reduction has been used to facilitate reduction and is said to decrease the rate of avascular necrosis [1–7]. Data from the literature, however, are not sufficient to support its efficiency or efficacy [8,9]. In the study by Kutlu and colleagues [10], preliminary traction did not affect the rate of avascular necrosis, even in young children. Femoral shortening is the alternative suggested by many investigators [11–20]. Today there is a tendency to recommend a one-stage procedure consisting of open reduction, femoral shortening, and pelvic osteotomy [21–27]. Other controversies exist about the best approach to performing an acetabular and femoral procedure, the maximum age at which treatment is worthwhile, and the type of acetabular correction indicated.

Indications

Closed reduction is the treatment of choice for most patients younger than 18 months of age. For children who are 18 to 24 months old, closed re-

Study performed at Hospital Pequeno Príncipe, Curitiba, PR, Brazil.
* Corresponding author. Rua Buenos Aires, 1020 Curitiba, PR 80250-070, Brazil.
E-mail address: eforlin@brturbo.com.br (E. Forlin).

duction is still possible; but the rate of failure and subsequent open reduction increases. In a study by Zionts and MacEwen [7], 60% of children older than walking age who were treated with closed reduction required a procedure for persistent acetabular dysplasia. After 24 months of age, most investigators recommend primary open reduction [22,25].

Some controversy exists about the minimum age at which an acetabular procedure can be performed. Because the potential with age for acetabular development is markedly diminished after the age of 18 months, Salter proposed his procedure be done after that age [1,4]. It can also be performed in patients who are 12 to 18 months old [28]. Others prefer to perform the open reduction and follow the development of the acetabulum [29,30]. Because many patients will later require an acetabular procedure, we believe it is easier to perform it at the time of the open reduction [1,2,4,21,22,25,27,31–36]. Another advantage of performing both procedures at the same time is that acetabuloplasty may add stability to the open reduction. As a principle, the more complete the correction of the deformities, the better the conditions for proper development of the hip joint [37]. The authors' indication for a concomitant acetabular procedure is for patients who are older than 18 months.

The grade of dislocation may influence the outcome [29]; but even for high dislocation or subluxation, the indication for most patients with untreated DDH may include the one-stage combined procedure.

Age limit for treatment

Although rare, some patients remain untreated at an older age. Opinions vary about the upper age limit when treatment may produce a worse end result (with a high risk of complications) than no treatment at all. Some investigators suggest that children less than the age of four years at operation had better results [4,38,39]. Mckay [40] found better results in children younger than age six years. In other studies, the age at operation varied from 6 to 15 years [6,17,19,22,41–43]. Reviewing 32 patients who had 44 hips treated with open reduction and Salter osteotomy and who ranged in age from 18 to 90 months, the authors did not find any correlation of the end result with age at reduction (Edilson Forlin, MD, Akira Ishida, MD, MSc, PhD, Carlo Milani, MD, MSc, PhD, unpublished data, 2005). For bilateral cases, the authors prefer to perform one side at each session.

As shown by the long-term study of Malvitz and Weinstein [8], however, for patients treated with closed reduction, the younger the patient is at the time of reduction, the better the clinical and the radiographic results. The same may also be said for open reduction. Because of the risk of complications such as avascular necrosis and stiffness, the surgeon and the parents must be aware of the risk for a poor end result, especially in older children. The decision to operate on patients older than 10 years should be made with caution. The authors do not recommend the procedure in bilateral cases after this age. It is important to inform the parents that the child may remain with some limp and restriction of mobility. If avascular necrosis occurs, a stiff joint can result.

Treatment options

Open reduction

Some of the factors we related in the pathoanatomy are fundamental to the operative treatment. It is important to address the psoas, capsule, and transverse acetabular ligament. The ligamentum teres femoris and the pulvinar may have to be resected. With femoral shortening, adductor tenotomy is not necessary. The limbus rarely needs to be everted.

The quality of the reduction is the main determinant of the final result. The femoral head needs to be well-seated, which can be assessed clinically by the palpation of the femoral head close to the medial aspect of the acetabulum. (There should be no free space.) The correct seating of the femoral head can be confirmed radiographically by the position of the capital femoral epiphysis deep in the acetabulum and whether Shenton's line is continuous. The surgeon must confirm that all obstacles are addressed. This is the most important part of the operation, and it should be carefully performed.

Femoral shortening

To pull the femoral head down and allow reduction without compression there are two options: (1) preliminary traction for two or three weeks and, (2) femoral shortening. In the past, traction was used for children younger than age 4 years, with good results [4,6,39,44–47]. To be effective, the traction should bring the femoral head to the joint level [3]. Several studies, however, failed to demonstrate the usefulness of traction and instead showed better results and lower rates of avascular necrosis with femoral shortening [12,14,18,19,22,26,27,43]. In the studies of Westin and colleagues [14] and Schoenecker and Strecker [16], a total of 86 hips were evaluated. Forty-eight were treated with traction and

38 with femoral shortening. The results were superior in the femoral shortening group. Avascular necrosis was seen in 31 hips, all of which were in the traction group.

Femoral shortening is preferred because it may be more effective in reducing the pressure at the joint, facilitating the reduction and decreasing the rate of avascular necrosis without need for long-term hospitalization.

There are several techniques for femoral osteotomy and fixation. The authors do not find that correction of valgus of the neck is necessary and prefer to perform the shortening at the proximal diaphysis, using a four-hole dynamic compression plate (Fig. 1A–C). It is simple and less risky than a trochanteric or subtrochanteric osteotomy with the use of an angled plate.

Acetabular procedure

Acetabular procedures may be divided into redirectional and acetabuloplasty. Redirectional osteotomy is represented by the Salter procedure. It covers anteriorly and laterally, although at the expense of posterior coverage. An advantage is some gain in the length of the lower limb. The disadvantages are the potential increase in the pressure on the femoral head and nerve injury. Also, there is a need for a secondary procedure to remove the k-wires. As mentioned earlier, many investigators recommend the procedure be performed after the age of 18 months [4,6,22,29,38,39,48–53], but in very unstable hips it can be performed earlier [28,54].

The acetabuloplasty is represented by the Pemberton procedure and its modifications, and by the

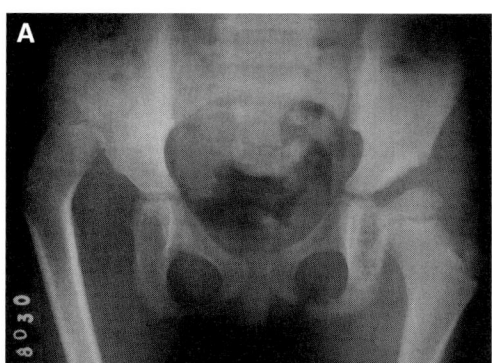
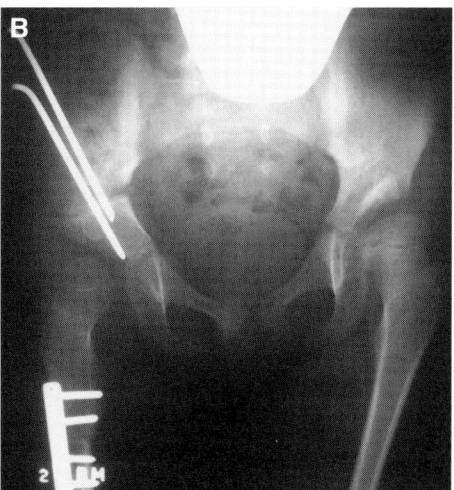
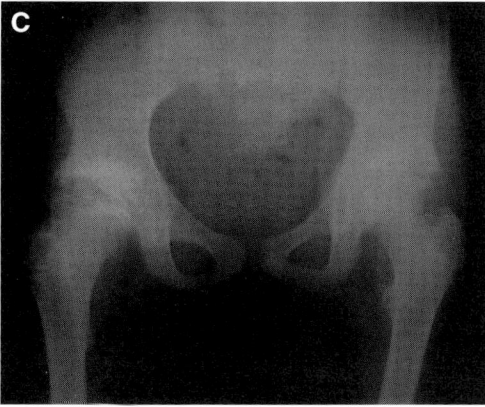

Fig. 1. (*A*) A six-year-old girl who has a high right dislocation and left-sided acetabular dysplasia. (*B*) Radiograph after open reduction femoral shortening and Salter osteotomy. (*C*) Same patient at age 11 years, showing good clinical result, with some irregularity of the joint from type II avascular necrosis.

Dega procedure [55–61]. These procedures change the shape of the acetabulum, and they can also have some effect on redirecting the acetabulum [59]. Both the Pemberton and Dega procedures allow greater correction of the acetabular dysplasia than Salter's osteotomy. Additionally, no internal fixation is needed The Pemberton procedure is believed to hinge at the triradiate cartilage; theoretically, it should be open for the procedure to be successful. Pemberton's original study in 1965 showed good results in children younger than 7 years [55]. Coleman [60] cautioned against the use of the osteotomy in children older than 6 years because of the decreased capacity of remodeling and the risk of redislocation. However, some studies report that the operation can be done later with good results [36,61]. One potential problem is to decrease the size of an already smaller acetabulum [24,62]. A complication associated with these procedures is premature closure of the triradiate cartilage [63–65]. The main risk is damage to the articular cartilage caused by wrong direction of the osteotomy. Overall, most techniques of acetabular osteotomy have a high rate of satisfactory results.

Operative procedure

Open reduction

The patient is placed supine on a radiolucent operating table. A support is placed under the lumbar spine to produce a 20° to 30° inclination. The anterolateral approach by way of a bikini incision allows good visualization, and the scar has an excellent cosmetic appearance. After the incision, the lateral femoral cutaneous nerve is identified and retracted medially. The interval between the tensor fascia and sartorius muscle is developed. The iliac crest apophyseal cartilage is split. The outer iliac wing is stripped subperiosteally with a sponge (the inner cortex is stripped later to avoid unnecessary bleeding) as distally as possible. Care must be taken at the level of the false acetabulum and in the space between the periosteum and the capsule. The rectus femoris muscles are reflected and the direct tendons are identified. They are transected and the reflected head is dissected because it is the guide of the acetabular border.

The capsule is well-exposed from posterolateral to medial. The iliopsoas muscle is identified medial to the joint and its tendoneous portion is divided. Before this point, it is preferable to identify the femoral nerve, anterior to the psoas, because it can be mistaken for the tendon.

The capsule is opened a few millimeters from its insertion at the acetabulum posterolateral to medial (the authors use scissors to carefully protect the articular cartilage). A second capsular incision is made in alignment with the femoral neck. The ligamentum teres can easily be identified after the first incision in the capsule. Its insertion is localized because it allows palpation of the transverse acetabular ligament. The ligamentum teres is resected, and the transverse acetabular ligament is divided. The pulvinar is resected, and it is verified that the medial part of the capsule was released. The anterolateral flap of the capsule, redundant and thick, is then resected (Fig. 2A). At this point, verification is made as to the possibility of reduction, the tension, and if there is excessive anteversion of the proximal femur. The anteversion is estimated with the knee flexed in the frontal plane.

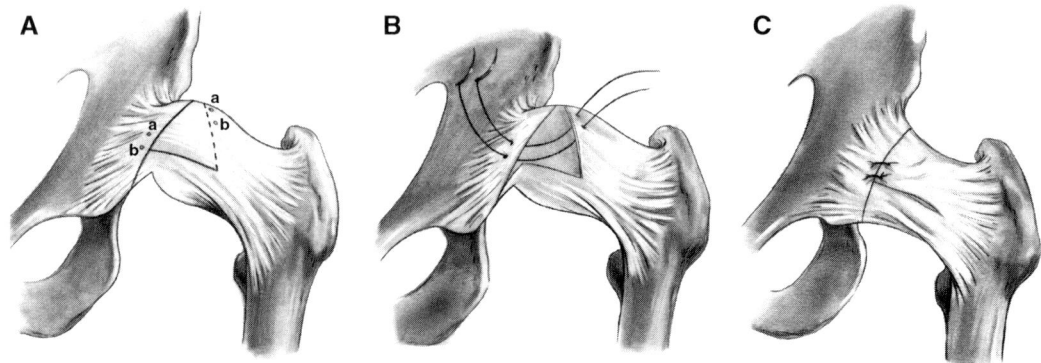

Fig. 2. The authors' approach to the capsule: (*A*) The anterolateral part of the capsule is resected. (*B*) The repair sutures are made before the acetabular osteotomy. (*C*) When the suture is tied, the tension provides more stability to the joint. The anteromedial part of the capsule is only released. No capsulorraphy is performed at this time.

Diaphyseal femoral shortening

The authors use a separate lateral incision, beginning just below the greater trochanter and extending distally 10 cm. The vastus lateralis is retracted anteriorly, and the femur exposed subperiosteally. A four-hole DCP plate is placed, and the proximal holes are made. The rotation is marked carefully. The authors usually avoid correcting all the anteversion. A 20° correction may be sufficient, especially if the Salter osteotomy is to be performed.

The initial femoral cut is done by using a power saw. To check the amount of shortening that is needed, the femoral head is reduced and the amount of overlap of the fragments is verified. Usually, this measure is approximately 2 cm. After resection of the segment, the plate is fixed proximally. The distal segment is then fixed after the derotation correction.

At this stage the reduction may be easily obtained without pressure. It is important to be sure that the femoral head is well-seated. Before performing the acetabular procedure, repair sutures of the capsulorrhaphy are placed. The authors use two or three sutures from the remaining anterolateral capsule to the acetabular rim, as medial as possible. The suture is tied only after the acetabular procedure is performed (Fig. 2B, C).

For the acetabuloplasty, the authors prefer the Dega procedure. The outer table of the ilium is exposed, ending at the sciatic notch, and a retractor is placed. The osteotomy is marked 1.5 cm superior to the labrum. Under the image intensifier control, the osteotome is directed toward the triradiate cartilage (Fig. 3). With the osteotome in place, the cut is completed anteriorly and posteriorly in a gently curved fashion. For most cases, a predominant anterior coverage is desirable; and the cut is performed more anteriorly (inner cortex). The authors have not found it necessary to extend the cuts back to the posterior notch. The segment removed from the femoral shaft is divided into two grafts. With the use of an osteotome or a laminar spreader, the osteotomy site is opened. The larger graft is inserted anteriorly and, when necessary, the smaller is inserted posterior to the larger. No internal fixation is needed. Finally, the capsule suture is tied. The position of the osteotomy and the reduction is checked by fluoroscopy or radiograph. The wound is closed and the child is placed in a one-and-a-half hip spica cast in a position of mild flexion, abduction, and internal rotation (20°–30°). The cast is maintained for six weeks. The child is then let out of the cast to regain motion. It is usually not necessary for the child to use abduction bracing after this time.

Results

There are few long-term studies of the functional and radiographic outcomes following the operative treatment of DDH. Most studies include several modalities of treatment, and it is difficult to analyze the influence of a specific factor or treatment. Also the effect of treatment of DDH can be assessed only after an adequate follow-up (skeletal maturity would be desirable), and most publications report short-term results. Few studies have reviewed the results with one-stage operation (open reduction, femoral shortening, and acetabular procedure).

Schoenecker and Strecker [16] compared traction with femoral shortening. In the first group (traction), there were 17 patients with 26 hips, and 8 patients with 13 hips were in the second group (femoral shortening). The mean age was lower in the first group (4 years, 8 months versus 5 years, 11 months in the second group). The length of follow-up was not similar (11 years versus 4 years). Group I had higher complications: 14 hips with avascular necrosis (none in group II), and 11 hips with redislocation (one in group II).

In the study by Klisic and colleagues [17] 144 patients underwent the one-stage operation. The Salter osteotomy was performed in 89 hips, Chiari osteotomy in 99 hips, and Pemberton osteotomy in 37 hips, the age at the time of the operation ranged from 7 to 15 years. The mean length of follow-up was 13 years (range, 9–24 years). The overall results were 66% good, 25% fair, and 10% poor.

Dimitriou and Cavadias [19] studied 67 hips in 52 patients. In 34 hips, a Salter osteotomy was performed. Age at the time of surgery ranged from 3 to 14 years. The mean length follow-up was

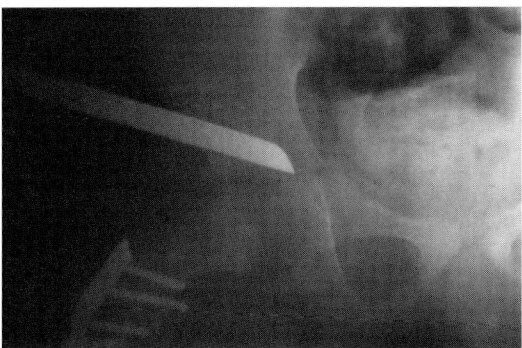

Fig. 3. A preoperative image is used to check reduction and the cut of the acetabulum in the Dega procedure.

11 years (range, 5–24 years). The results showed 53 hips as excellent, 13 as good, and 1 as fair. There were two cases of avascular necrosis [20].

Galpin and colleagues [22] reported on 25 patients who had 33 treated hips. Twenty-one had an associated acetabular procedure. Of the 19 hips that underwent an associated Salter osteotomy, 14 hips had a good result, four a fair, and one a poor result. The complications were three redislocations, two stiffness, three unstable hips, and one avascular necrosis.

Olney, Latz, and Asher [23] reviewed the results of combined one-stage procedure in 18 hips of 13 patients. The average age at the time the surgery was 29 months (range, 15–117 months) and the mean length of follow-up was 43 months. The acetabular procedure was the Pemberton osteotomy. Results showed all with good outcomes (16 Severin class IA and 2 class IIA). Avascular necrosis developed in one patient and no patient required a secondary procedure.

Ryan and colleagues [26] reviewed the results in 25 hips of 18 patients. There were 17 acetabular procedures. The age at the time of surgery ranged from 3 to 9 years. Eighteen hips had an excellent or good result at a mean follow-up of 10.5 years. Although avascular necrosis was observed in 11 hips, only four developed severe deformity. They recommended the procedure for patients from 3 to 10 years of age.

Böhm and Brzuske [29] reviewed 61 patients who had 73 Salter osteotomies and a follow-up ranging from 26 to 35 years. Only three hips underwent a combined one-stage procedure. Fifty-nine were classified as good results by Severin classification (Fig. 4A–C) [65]. Clinical outcome was related to the grade of dislocation preoperatively, the postoperative grade of dysplasia, the grade of avascular necrosis, and the technique of reduction.

The authors reviewed 32 children who had 44 hips treated with open reduction and Salter osteotomy (Forlin et al, in preparation, 2005). Twenty-six hips had preliminary skeletal traction and 18 hips had a concomitant femoral shortening. There were 23 good, 12 fair, and 9 poor results. Ten hips had avascular necrosis and four had redislocation. An initial satis-

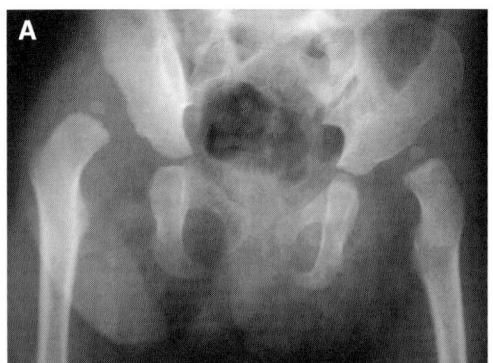
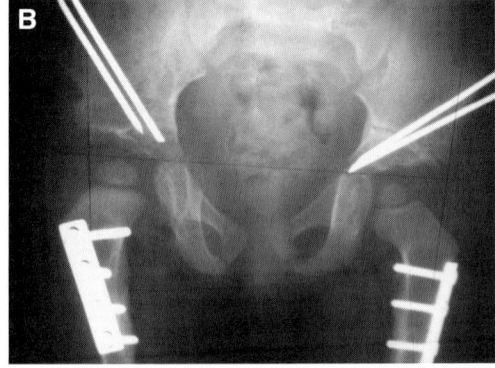
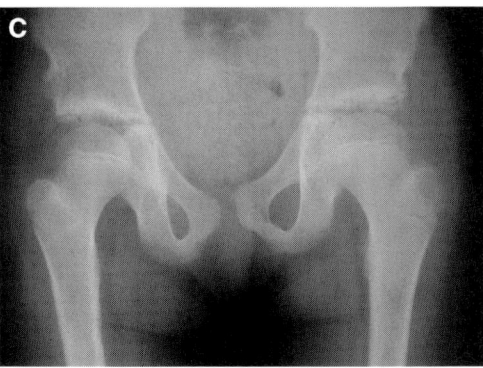

Fig. 4. A two-and-one-half year old girl who has a bilateral dislocation: (*A*) preoperative radiograph, (*B*) postoperatively after a bilateral procedure, and (*C*) last radiograph at age 9 years, showing result with Severin class IA and good clinical outcome.

factory reduction and osteotomy were related with better result. Redislocation was more common in the traction group, but there was no difference in the rate of avascular necrosis in the traction group compared with the femoral shortening group (in the past, the authors employed skeletal traction). In another study from the same institution, the authors reviewed 24 hips of 20 patients treated after the age of 4 years (range, 4 to 12 years). The mean length of follow-up was 5 years. Seventy percent of the hips had an excellent or good result (Severin IA, IB, and II) (see Fig. 4A–C). Avascular necrosis was seen in six hips. Results were related to age at the time of operation; worse outcomes were found in patients older than seven years at the time of the operation.

From the literature, the rate of good results with the one-stage combined procedure reaches 70% to 80% at short-term follow-up (this index may drop at long-term review). Most investigators recommend that the open reduction be done with an associated acetabular procedure. Femoral shortening may be necessary in children under the age of 3 years when, at the time of the reduction, there is tension or difficulty in lowering the femoral head. After the age of 3 years, femoral shortening is required for almost all patients.

Complications

Avascular necrosis

The rate of avascular necrosis in older children seems to be comparable to that in young children. If considering only the clinically relevant cases of avascular necrosis, the rate is less than 10%. One difficulty in comparing the studies is the criteria to classify avascular necrosis. Salter's criteria seem broad, because even a well-developed joint with a regular but larger femoral head can be classified as avascular necrosis (Fig. 5A–C). Using the Kalamchi and MacEwen [66] classification, the authors found that the type I pattern may have no clinical consequence. Avascular necrosis may be related to the

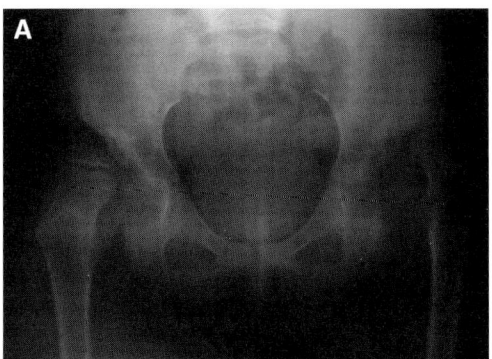
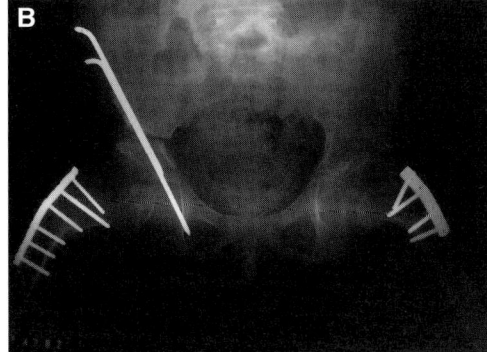
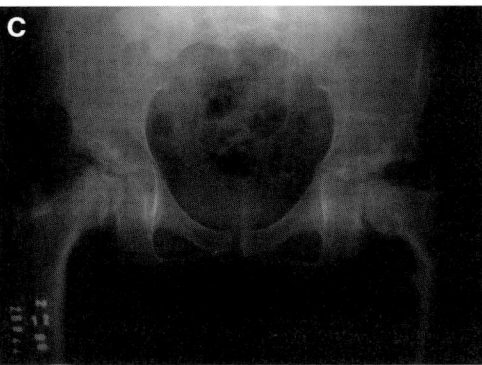

Fig. 5. (*A*) A seven-and-one-half year old girl who has bilateral dislocation. (*B*) Postoperative radiograph after a bilateral combined one-stage procedure with Salter osteotomy. (*C*) At age 13 years, the hips were centered but grade I avascular necrosis is observed bilaterally. The function is very good on both sides.

open reduction (Salter). The lesion of the proximal femoral growth plate may result in a limb-length discrepancy. Severe cases of avascular necrosis may cause pain and marked limitation of motion or even permanent stiffness (Fig. 6A–D).

Redislocation

Redislocation in the early postoperative period may have several causes. The possibilities are nonconcentric reduction because of failure to release all obstacles, femoral malrotation, insufficient acetabular coverage, capsular loosing, and inappropriate immobilization. In cases of redislocation, the authors recommend evaluation and arthrograms under general anesthesia to assess the factors that can obstruct the reduction. If concentric and stable reduction is possible, a few weeks of continued immobilization in a cast is indicated. In cases of impending instability, an operative revision is indicated.

Stiffness

The authors have seen some patients developed a stiff hip without avascular necrosis. It may represent some insult to the articular cartilage or intra-articular scar and fibrosis similar to chondrolysis. In these cases, the authors start the patient on physical therapy and traction. If restriction of motion remains, manipulation under general anesthesia is tried. Usually, reasonable mobility is obtained at the manipulation. However, range of motion decreases at follow-up. The indication for a surgical debridement is not well-established.

Residual dysplasia

Some patients will remain with residual dysplasia at an older age. It is important to follow the patients to skeletal maturity to verify acetabular development and maintenance of the concentric position

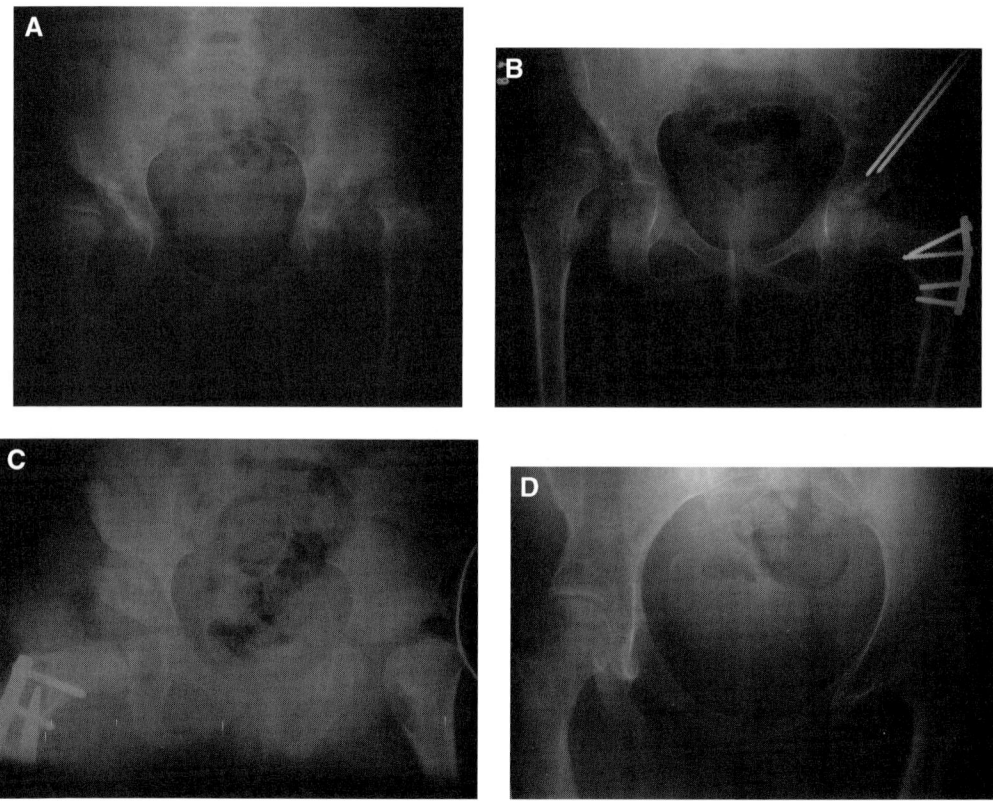

Fig. 6. (*A*) A five-year-old girl who has a bilateral dislocation. (*B*) After an one-stage combined procedure (with Salter osteotomy) at left side. (*C*) Six months postoperatively avascular necrosis grade IV of Kalamchi and MacEwen is seen. Even with the poor outcome at the left side, the patient underwent one-stage procedure (with Pemberton) on the right hip. (*D*) Final result. The left side has an ankylosis. Right hip showed excellent clinical and radiographic outcome.

(Fig. 7A–E). The presence of a sclerotic triangle at the support area in the acetabulum, the disruption of Shenton's line, the increase of the acetabular angle, and decrease of a center edge angle may indicate the development of abnormal pressure resulting from mechanical malfunction. Long-term studies have demonstrated that dysplasia tends to lead to a subluxation and degenerative changes in early adulthood [8,29].

Osteoarthritis

When well-performed, the one-stage procedure recreates a nearly normal hip anatomy and allows development of hip function. Irregularity of the joint may produce osteoarthrosis at long-term follow-up. More pronounced deformity and avascular necrosis would lead to early degenerative changes. Even hips that present with a good joint appearance may de-

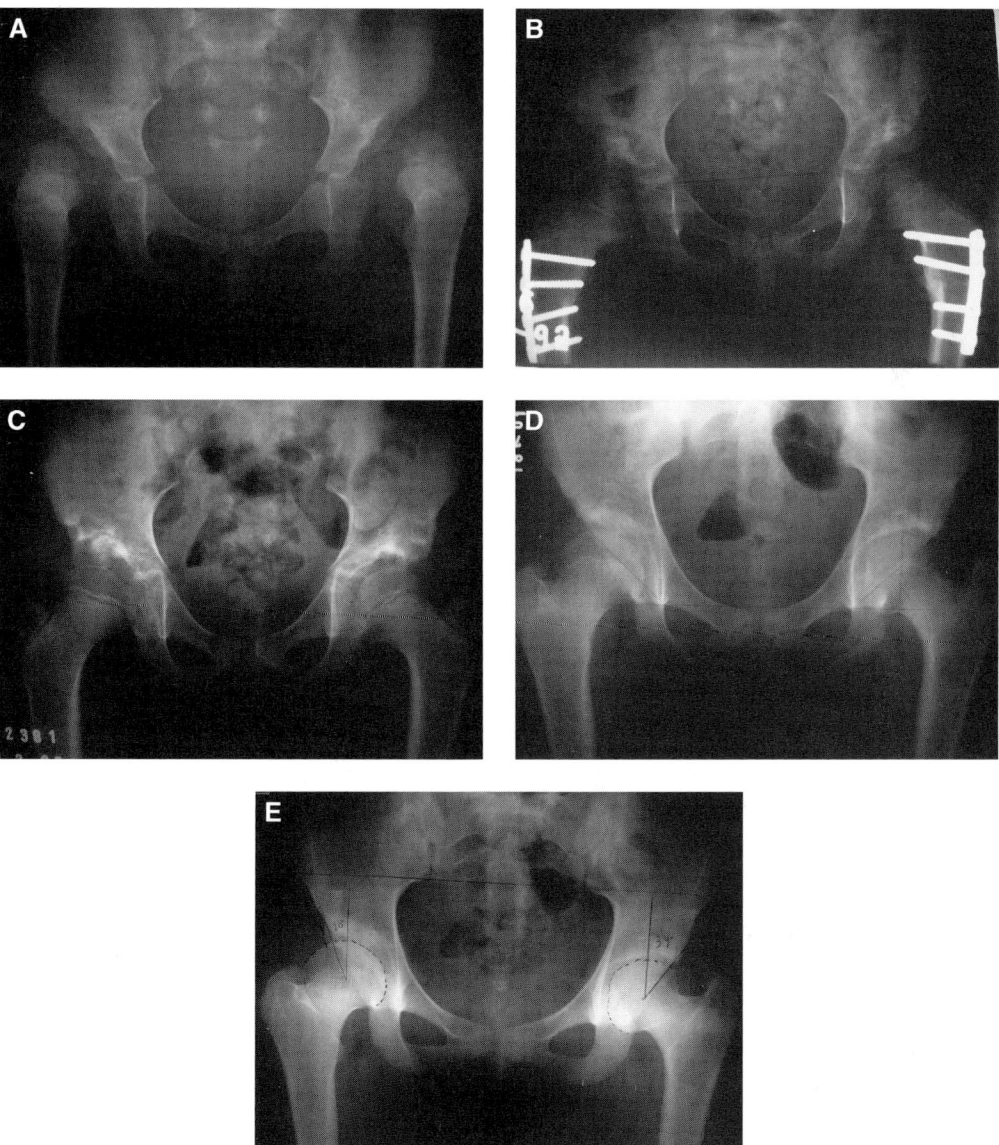

Fig. 7. (*A*) A two-and-one-half year-old girl who has bilateral dislocation. (*B*) Six months after one-stage combined procedure on the left side and three months after the same procedure on the right side. (*C*) At the age of 8 years: although reduced, acetabular dysplasia can be recognized on the right side. (*D*) At age 12 years, acetabular dysplasia is still persistent. (*E*) Final result at age 15 years: hip is well-centered but mild dysplasia persists at right hip.

velop osteoarthritis. Kalamchi and MacEwen [66] showed late disturbance of growth following treatment of DDH. The same was observed by Malvitz and Weinstein [8], but it was not directly correlated with the clinical function at a 30-year follow-up. In a long-term study, Böhm and Brzuske [29] found that 65% of the hips had some degree of radiographic osteoarthrosis, but the rate did not changed significantly from 25 to 30 years of follow-up.

Summary

The authors believe that in the older child who has untreated DDH, the one-stage procedure—consisting of open reduction, femoral shortening, and pelvic osteotomy—yields satisfactory results. The complex pathologic anatomy must be recognized and corrected. It is a demanding procedure and more challenging technically than a staged procedure; but it can be done safely and effectively, providing good conditions for a satisfactory development of the hip joint.

Acknowledgments

The authors thank Andre B. Ducci, for the illustrations and Carla M. Forlin for the help with the English.

References

[1] Salter RB. Innominate osteotomy in the treatment of congenital dislocation and subluxation of the hip. J Bone Joint Surg Br 1961;43:518–39.

[2] Salter RB, Kostuik J, Dallas S. Avascular necrosis of the femoral head as a complication of treatment for congenital dislocation of the hip in young children: a clinical and experimental investigation. Can J Surg 1969;12:44–61.

[3] Gage JR, Winter RB. Avascular necrosis of the capital femoral epiphysis as a complication of closed reduction of congenital dislocation of the hip: a critical review of twenty years experience at Gillette Children's Hospital. J Bone Joint Surg Am 1971;54:373–88.

[4] Salter RB, Dubos JP. The first fifteen years' personal experience with innominate osteotomy in treatment of congenital dislocation of the hip in young children. Clin Orthop 1974;98:72–103.

[5] Weiner DS, Hoyt WAJ, O'Dell HW. Congenital dislocation of the hip. The relationship of premanipulation traction and age to avascular necrosis of the femoral head. J Bone Joint Surg Am 1977;54:306–11.

[6] Shih J, Chen H, Liu H. Interim follow-up studies of innominate osteotomy for congenital dislocation of the hip. Clin Orthop 1980;152:261–5.

[7] Zionts LE, MacEwen GD. Treatment of congenital dislocation of the hip in children between the ages of one and three years. J Bone Joint Surg Am 1986;68: 829–46.

[8] Malvitz TA, Weinstein SL. Closed reduction for congenital dysplasia of the hip: functional and radiographic results after an average of thirty years. J Bone Joint Surg Am 1994;76:1777–92.

[9] Weinstein SL. Traction in developmental dislocation of the hip: is its use justified? Clin Orthop 1997;338: 79–85.

[10] Kutlu A, Ayata C, Ogun TC, et al. Preliminary traction as a single determinant of avascular necrosis in developmental dislocation of the hip. J Pediatr Orthop 2000;20(5):579–84.

[11] Leveuf J. Results of the open reduction of "true" congenital luxation of the hip. J Bone Joint Surg Am 1948;309:875–82.

[12] Ashley RK, Larsen LJ, James PM. Reduction of dislocation of the hip in older children. J Bone Joint Surg Am 1972;54(A):545–50.

[13] Browne RS. The management of late diagnosed congenital dislocation and subluxation of the hip. With special reference to femoral shortening. J Bone Joint Surg Br 1979;61:7–12.

[14] Westin GW, Dallas TG, Watanabe BM, et al. Skeletal traction vs. femoral shortening in treatment of older children with congenital hip dislocation. Jsr J Med Sci 1980;16:318–22.

[15] Gallien R, Bertin D, Lirette R. Salter procedure in congenital dislocation of the hip. J Pediatr Orthop 1984;4:427–30.

[16] Schoenecker PL, Strecker WB. Congenital dislocation of the hip in children. Comparison of the effects of femoral shortening and of skeletal traction in treatment. J Bone and Joint Surg Am 1984;66:21–7.

[17] Klisic P, Jankovic L, Basara V. Long-term results of combined operative reduction of the hip in older children. J Pediatr Orthop 1988;8:532–4.

[18] Shih C, Shih H. One-stage combined operation of congenital dislocation of the hips in older children. J Pediatr Orthop 1988;8:535–9.

[19] Dimitriou JK, Cavadias AX. One-stage surgical procedure for congenital dislocation of the hip in older children: long-term results. Clin Orthop 1989;246: 30–8.

[20] Killian G, Hoffmann EB. One stage treatment of congenital dislocation of the hip in older children. In Orthopaedic Proceedings: South African Orthopaedic Association. J Bone Joint Surg Br 1997; 79(4S) Supplement:444.

[21] Klisic P, Jankovic L. Combined procedure of open reduction and shortening of the femur in treatment of congenital dislocation of the hips in older children. Clin Orthop 1976;119:60–9.

[22] Galpin RD, Roach JW, Wenger DR, et al. One-stage treatment of congenital dislocation of the hip in older

[22] children, including femoral shortening. J Bone Joint Surg Am 1989;71:734–41.
[23] Olney B, Latz K, Asher M. Treatment of hip dysplasia in older children with a combined one-stage procedure. Clin Orthop 1998;347:215–23.
[24] Grudziak JS, Labaziewicz L, Kruczynski J, et al. Combined one-staged open reduction, femoral osteotomy, and Dega pelvic osteotomy for developmental dysplasia of the hip. J Pediatr Orthop 1993;13:680.
[25] Weinstein LS, Mubarak JS, Wenger RD. Developmental hip dysplasia and dislocation: part II. J Bone Joint Surg Am 2003;85:2024–35.
[26] Ryan MG, Johnson LO, Quanbeck DS, et al. One-stage treatment of congenital dislocation of the hip in children three to ten years old: functional and radiographic results. J Bone Joint Surg Am 1998;80:336–44.
[27] Karakas ES, Baktir A, Argun M, et al. One-stage treatment of congenital dislocation of the hip in older children. J Pediatr Orthop 1995;15:330–6.
[28] Lin CJ, Lin YT, Laika A. Intraoperative instability for developmental dysplasia of the hip in children 12 to 18 months of age as a guide to Salter osteotomy. J Pediatr Orthop 2000;20(5):575–8.
[29] Böhm P, Brzuske A. Salter innominate osteotomy for the treatment of developmental dysplasia of the hip in children. Results of seventy-three consecutive osteotomies after twenty-six to thirty-five years of follow-up. J Bone Joint Surg Am 2002;84(2):178–86.
[30] Nakamura M, Matsunaga S, Yoshino S, et al. Long-term result of combination of open reduction and femoral derotation varus osteotomy with shortening for developmental dislocation of the hip. J Pediatr Orthop B 2004;13(4):248–53.
[31] Salter RB. Role of innominate osteotomy in the treatment of congenital dislocation and subluxation of the hip in the older child. J Bone Joint Surg Am 1966;48:1413–39.
[32] Haidar RK, Jones RS, Vergroesen DA, et al. Simultaneous open reduction and Salter innominate osteotomy for developmental dysplasia of the hip. J Bone Joint Surg Br 1996;78:471–6.
[33] Huang SC, Wang JH. A comparative study of non-operative versus operative treatment of developmental dysplasia of the hip in patients of walking age. J Pediatr Orthop 1997;17(2):181–8.
[34] Nattrass GR, DelBello DA, Watts HG, et al. Concurrent Salter innominate osteotomy at the time of open reduction of congenital dislocation of the hip. J Bone Joint Surg Br 2000;82(4S, Suppl II):154.
[35] Ito H, Ooura H, Kobayashi M, et al. Middle-term results of Salter innominate osteotomy. Clin Orthop Relat Res 2001;387:156–64.
[36] Wada A, Fujii T, Takamura K, et al. Pemberton osteotomy for developmental dysplasia of the hip in older children. J Pediatr Orthop 2003;23(4):508–13.
[37] Angliss R, Fujii G, Pickvance E, et al. Surgical treatment of late developmental displacement of the hip. Results after 33 years. J Bone Joint Surg Br 2005;87(3):384–94.
[38] Roth A, Gibson DA, Hall JE. The experience of five surgeons with innominate osteotomy in the treatment of congenital dislocation and subluxation of the hip. Clin Orthop 1974;98:178–82.
[39] Barrett WP, Staheli LT, Chew DE. The effectiveness of the Salter innominate osteotomy in the treatment of congenital dislocation of the hip. J Bone Joint Surg Am 1986;68:79–87.
[40] Mckay DW. A comparison of the innominate and the pericapsular osteotomy in the treatment of congenital dislocation of the hip. Clin Orthop 1974;98:124–32.
[41] Herold HZ, Daniel D. Reduction of neglected congenital dislocation of the hip in children over the age of six years. J Bone Joint Surg Br 1979;61(1):1–6.
[42] Marafioti RL, Westin GW. Factors influencing the results of acetabuloplasty in children. J Bone Joint Surg Am 1980;62:765–9.
[43] Williamson DM, Glover SD, Benson MKDA. Congenital dislocation of the hip presenting after the age of three years. A long-term review. J Bone Joint Surg Br 1989;71(5):745–51.
[44] Lalonde DF, Frick SL, Wenger DR. Surgical correction of residual hip dysplasia in two pediatric age-groups. J Bone Joint Surg Am 2002;84:1148–56.
[45] Greco Jr CH. The use of skeletal traction as a preliminary procedure in the treatment of early congenital dislocation of the hip. J Bone Joint Surg Am 1939;21:353–72.
[46] Waters P, Kurica K, Hall J, et al. Salter innominate osteotomies in congenital dislocation of the hip. J Pediatr Orthop 1988;8:650–5.
[47] Daoud A, Saighi-Bououina A. Congenital dislocation of the hip in the older child: the effectiveness of overhead traction. J Bone Joint Surg Am 1996;78(1):30–4.
[48] Crelin RQ. Innominate osteotomy for congenital dislocation and subluxation of the hip: a follow-up study. Clin Orthop 1974;98:171–7.
[49] Denton JR, Ryder CT. Radiographic follow-up of Salter innominate osteotomy for congenital dysplasia of the hip. Clin Orthop 1974;98:210–3.
[50] Gallien R, Bertin D, Lirette R. Salter procedure in congenital dislocation of the hip. J Pediatr Orthop 1984;4:427–30.
[51] Hansson G, Althoff B, Bylund P, et al. The Swedish experience with Salter's innominate osteotomies in the treatment of congenital subluxation and dislocation of the hip. J Pediatr Orthop 1990;10:159–62.
[52] Zadeh HG, Catterall A, Hashemi-Nejad A, et al. Test of stability as an aid to decide the need for osteotomy in association with open reduction in developmental dysplasia of the hip: a long-term review. J Bone Joint Surg Br 2000;82(1):17–27.
[53] Ito H, Ooura H, Kobayashi M, et al. Middle-term results of Salter innominate osteotomy. Clin Orthop 2001;387:156–64.
[54] Uyttendaele D, Burssens P, Mortele H, et al. Open reduction and innominate osteotomy in the treatment of C.D.H. between 15 and 18 months of age. Acta Orthop Belg 1990;56:251–6.

[55] Pemberton PA. Pericapsular osteotomy of the ilium for treatment of congenital subluxation and dislocation of the hip. J Bone Joint Surg Am 1965;47:65–86.

[56] Dega W. Schwierigkeiten in der chirurgischen reposition der veralteten kongenitalen subluxation des hüftgelenkes bei Kindern. Beitrage zur Orthopadie und Traumatologie 1964;11:642–7.

[57] Dega W. Selection of surgical methods in the treatment of congenital dislocation of the hip in children. Chir Narzadow Ruchu Ortop Pol 1969;34:357–66.

[58] Dega W. Transiliac osteotomy in the treatment of congenital hip dysplasia. Chir Narzadow Ruchu Ortop Pol 1974;39:601–13.

[59] Grudziak SJ, Ward TW. Dega osteotomy for the treatment of congenital dysplasia of the hip. J Bone Joint Surg Am 2001;83:845–54.

[60] Coleman SS. The incomplete pericapsular (Pemberton) and innominate (Salter) osteotomies. Clin Orthop 1974;98:116–23.

[61] Vedantam R, Capelli AM, Schoenecker P. Pemberton osteotomy for developmental dysplasia of the hip in older children. J Pediatr Orthop 1998;18(2):254–8.

[62] Slomczykowski M, Mackenzie WG, Stern G, et al. Acetabular volume. J Pediatr Orthop 1998;18(5):657–61.

[63] Leet AI, Mackenzie WG, Szoke G, et al. Injury to the growth plate after Pemberton osteotomy. J Bone Joint Surg Am 1999;81:169–76.

[64] Plaster RL, Schoenecker PL, Capelli AM. Premature closure of the triradiate cartilage: a potential complication of pericapsular acetabuloplasty. J Pediatr Orthop 1991;11:676–8.

[65] Severin E. Contribution to the knowledge of congenital dislocation of the hip joint. Late results of closed reduction and arthrographic studies of recent cases. Acta Chir Scand 1941;(Suppl):63.

[66] Kalamchi A, MacEwen GD. Avascular necrosis following treatment of congenital dislocation of the hip. J Bone Joint Surg Am 1980;62:876–88.

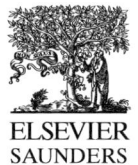

Treatment of Late Dysplasia with Ganz Osteotomy

Daniel J. Sucato, MD, MS

*Texas Scottish Rite Hospital for Children, Department of Orthopaedic Surgery,
University of Texas at Southwestern Medical Center, 2222 Welborn Street, Dallas, TX 75219, USA*

Hip dysplasia describes a wide spectrum of disease and is the leading cause of early osteoarthritis of the hip requiring reconstruction [1,2]. Patients may present many years following nonoperative treatment (ie, Pavlik harness) or operative treatment, including previous open reduction or reorientation of the acetabulum. Silent dysplasia may occur in the patient who has had no previous identification of hip pathology and presents in the adolescent or young adult. The age at which presentation occurs usually inversely depends on the severity of the disease. That is, patients who present at a younger age usually have more severe dysplasia, whereas those who have less severe dysplasia present in the adult age group. Pain is usually the presenting symptom and is most often lateral abductor fatigue pain or anterior groin pain. Previous osteotomies have relied on reorientation of the acetabulum, which have been more distant to the point of deformity (acetabulum). The Ganz periacetabular osteotomy was first described in 1988 and has significantly changed or improved on the previous reorientation procedures in that the osteotomy lines are close to the acetabulum [3]. The Ganz periacetabular osteotomy is believed to improve the long-term health of the hip and to prevent or delay early osteoarthritis to avoid reconstruction and morbidity.

This article briefly overviews hip dysplasia and its biomechanical and morphologic abnormalities, outlines the analysis of each patient, addresses the technical aspects of the Ganz periacetabular osteotomy, and finally describes the outcome reports using this procedure.

E-mail address: Dan.Sucato@tsrh.org

Hip dysplasia

Hip dysplasia refers to the abnormal acetabular morphology in which the acetabular slope is accentuated, leading to lateralization of the hip joint center, increased acetabular index of the weightbearing zone, an increased lateral center edge angle (Fig. 1), and an increased ventral central edge angle as seen on the false-profile view. These radiographic abnormalities describe the morphologic changes of the acetabulum and its relationship to the femoral head. These radiographic changes can be analyzed biomechanically, leading to an increased stress across the hip. Because stress equals force divided by area, this stress can be divided into these two components. The joint reaction force is increased, because the hip joint is generally lateralized compared with the opposite hip. This increases the length of the body moment arm, which in single stance results in a greater abductor muscle force to prevent the opposite pelvis from dropping (Trendelenburg sign and gait). The simple mathematic analysis demonstrates that a lateralization of the hip joint center by 2 cm in a 150-pound patient leads to an increase of the joint reaction force by 75 pounds with each step. In addition to the increase in force, the surface area is decreased, because the weightbearing zone of the acetabulum is significantly decreased with the obliquity of the acetabulum in the AP view and the lateral view. This decreased area similarly increases the stress across the hip joint. With acetabular dysplasia, vector analysis demonstrates that the sheer forces from an oblique acetabulum lead to further lateralization of the hip joint center and further displacement with time, especially as the articular cartilage degenerates. The biomechanical situation, even in mild dysplasia, can result in early osteoarthritis.

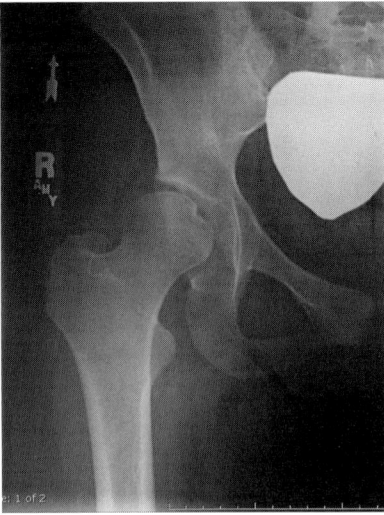

Fig. 1. An AP radiograph demonstrating the findings of hip dysplasia with an oblique sourcil (increased acetabular index of the weightbearing zone), decreased lateral coverage of the femoral head by the acetabulum (increased lateral center edge angle), lateralization of the hip joint center with subluxation (break in Shenton's line), and decreased anterior coverage of the femoral head by the acetabulum.

This also leads to the typical appearance of the patient during gait in which a Trendelenburg lurch is seen with the patient trying to center their body weight over the femoral head to decrease the adduction moment.

In addition to the bony abnormalities, hip dysplasia may lead to soft tissue injury. The acetabular labrum is the rim of soft tissue surrounding the acetabulum. With acetabular dysplasia, decreased surface area for weightbearing results, requiring the labrum to support the femoral head. Labral pathology is usually the result of overload and can result in early degeneration, labral tears, and the acetabular rim syndrome [4], which demonstrates avulsion of the acetabulum with excess stress across the labrum. Abnormalities of the labrum should be fully identified before any reorientation procedure of the acetabulum [5–7]. In general, the labral pathology then should be addressed at the time of the surgical reorientation procedure of the acetabulum.

History and physical examination

The history of the patient who presents with late hip dysplasia should identify any previous history of hip pathology. Many times patients present with a long history of hip pain and previous treatment. The patients who have a history of developmental dysplasia of the hip (DDH) who were treated with nonoperative methods such as Pavlik harness, Frejka pillow, double diapering, and abduction splint should be identified. More severe dysplasia may have been treated with a closed reduction with hip spica casting, or often in open reduction with an additional acetabular procedure, capsulorrhaphy, and femoral shortening. These patients often have acetabular dysplasia when they are young, and these patients are more challenging when planning surgical treatment during the adolescent period because of previous surgery, which leaves the patient with scarring and distortion of the pelvic anatomy. These patients present with acetabular dysplasia more often at an earlier age with more severe symptoms and radiographic findings. Acetabular dysplasia without previous operative intervention results in delay of the onset of symptoms until the patient's third or fourth decade of life (Fig. 2).

Once the previous history has been established, the current symptoms should be identified fully. The initial symptom a patient presents with in adolescent or adult hip dysplasia is usually lateral hip pain caused by the abductor muscle fatigue. This should be identified and differentiated from anterior groin pain, which is most often from symptoms coming directly from the hip joint itself. These symptoms can be caused by joint overload or labral pathology. Patients who have labral pathology often describe catching or locking symptoms or a popping sensation in their hip joint. Often parents of the adolescent patient or spouses of adult patients describe a more significant abductor lurch at the end of the day as the patient fatigues.

The physical examination should begin with an examination of the patient's gait. The adolescent patient often tries to demonstrate a more normal walking pattern, and walking a long hallway while conversing with a patient often brings out their true gait pattern. Those who have mild dysplasia may not demonstrate an initial Trendelenburg sign or gait, but with prolonged walking this may occur. The Trendelenburg sign (dropping of the contralateral pelvis in single limb stance) is another identification of relative abductor muscle weakness. This may require examination multiple times to bring this out as the patient's abductor muscles fatigue.

The patient then should be examined in the supine position to assess the range of motion of their hip. Generally patients have overall good motion unless there is severe subluxation of the hip in which abduction may be limited. In addition, any significant labral pathology may result in pain, especially with

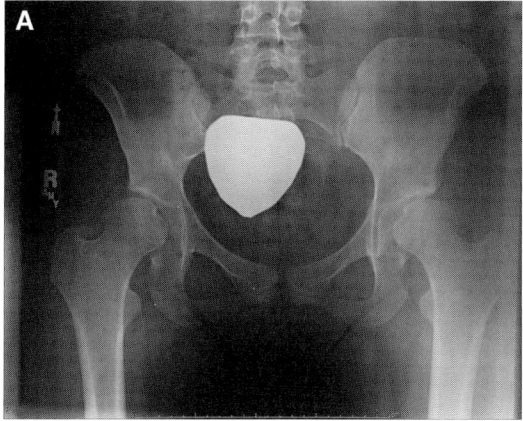
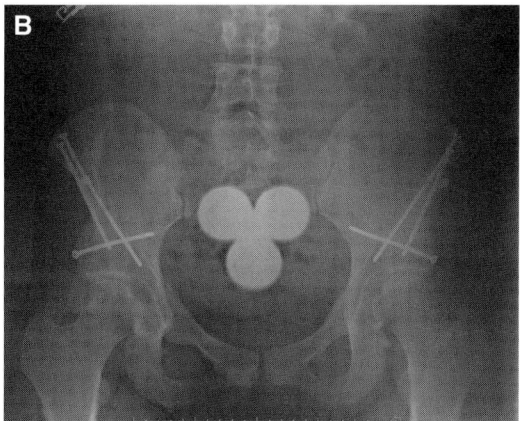

Fig. 2. Delayed presentation of acetabular dysplasia. (*A*) AP radiograph of a 32-year-old woman who presented with bilateral grouping pain beginning 1 year ago. The symptoms are fairly mild but constant and the radiographs demonstrate mild acetabular dysplasia without distortion of the pelvis from previous surgical treatment. (*B*) The postoperative radiograph following staged Bernese periacetabular osteotomies. Restoration of a horizontal sourcil is demonstrated with excellent lateral hip coverage. The patient is asymptomatic following her surgery.

flexion. The impingement test is sensitive for labral pathology. This test is done with flexion, adduction, and internal rotation of the hip. The more severe labral pathology may demonstrate pain at more mild ranges of motion, whereas mild dysplasia may require excessive flexion, adduction, and internal rotation, depending on symptoms. The instability test is performed with extension, abduction, and external rotation and often is believed to be caused by the hip having some instability anteriorly. This test is somewhat difficult to perform and the author has not found it terribly useful. A good neurologic examination is important to document the motor and sensory examination, especially before surgery and in the patient who has an underlying diagnosis.

The imaging modalities used for patients who have hip dysplasia include a standing anteroposterior (AP) pelvis radiograph without any rotation (see Fig. 1). This is used to assess the acetabular index of the weightbearing zone (AIWB) and the lateral center edge angle (LCEA). This radiograph also should be analyzed to tell whether the hip is subluxated (break in Shenton's line), because this is an important prognostic parameter leading to a poor outcome [1]. The abduction internal rotation (AIR) is used to assess whether the femoral head reduces concentrically into the acetabulum (Fig. 3). When concentric reduction is seen, a reorientation of the acetabulum procedure is indicated. The AIR view is difficult to obtain in a symptomatic patient, often necessitating positioning by the treating physician or member of the treating team. Because acetabular dysplasia is a three-dimensional (3-D) deformity, a false-profile radiograph is used to assess the ventral center edge angle (VCEA) (Fig. 4). This radiograph is performed aligning the radiograph beam perpendicular to the patient when they are standing in the lateral position. The hip that is not imaged then is rotated 25° out of plane to allow for full visualization of the opposite acetabulum. The VCEA is measured in a similar manner as the LCEA and should be greater than 20° to 25° on the false-profile radiograph.

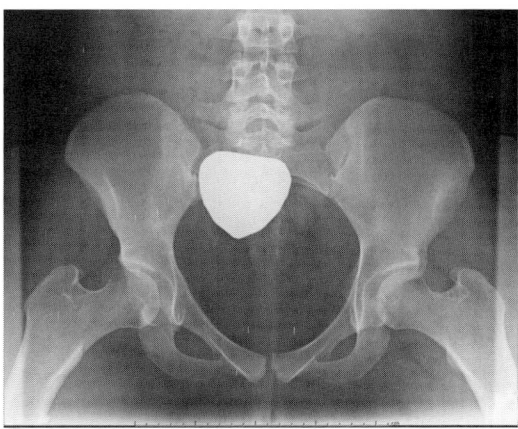

Fig. 3. The abduction internal rotation view (AIR) demonstrates that both femoral heads reduce concentrically into the acetabulum, a prerequisite for a reorientation procedure.

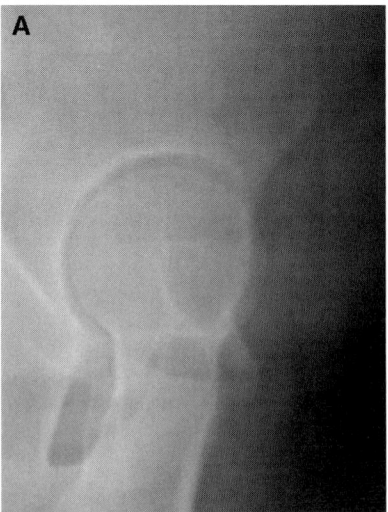
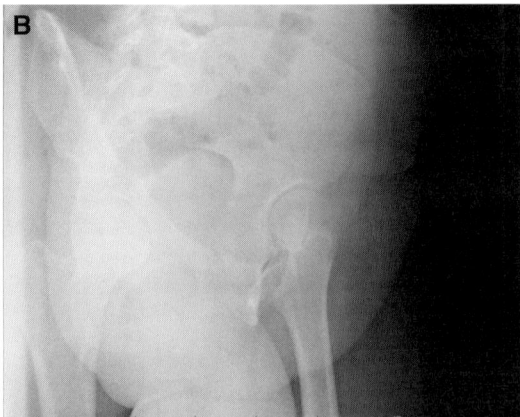

Fig. 4. The false-profile radiograph. (*A*) A normal false-profile radiograph demonstrating a normal ventral center edge angle. (*B*) A false-profile radiograph of a patient who had hip dysplasia demonstrating significant uncovering of the femoral head by the acetabulum anteriorly.

More advanced imaging studies are usually unnecessary in the patient who presents late with acetabular dysplasia. These can include a computed tomography (CT) examination with 3-D reconstruction to assess the morphology of the acetabulum and the sphericity of the femoral head. The author has found the CT scan to be most useful when the patients are skeletally immature when the osseous structures of the acetabulum are not fully defined on plain radiograph. MRI arthrography often is indicated in the older patient to fully assess articular cartilage pathology and in those patients who have a positive impingement sign to assess labral pathology. Leunig analyzed 14 adult patients who had symptomatic hip dysplasia and demonstrated labral tears in 9, enlargement of the labrum in 12, and ganglion formation in 10 [7]. Although this is an advanced imaging study, it is certainly becoming more routine, and the author has found it to be useful in helping predict those patients who will have a good outcome, because severe labral pathology and articular cartilage degeneration often lead to a poor prognosis [8]. The delayed gadolinium-enhanced magnetic imaging of cartilage (dGEMRIC) is a more recent technique that analyzes the changes in glycosaminoglycan in femoral and acetabular articular cartilage. Kim and colleagues demonstrated that the dGEMRIC index correlated with pain and the lateral center edge index and the severity of the dysplasia [9].

Once the diagnosis of hip dysplasia is identified, those patients who have pain are best treated with reorientation of the acetabulum to (1) medialize the hip joint (ultimately decreasing the hip joint reaction forces), and (2) horizontalize the sourcil in the AP and false profile views (increasing the weightbearing surface area). The indications for the Ganz periacetabular osteotomy are those patients who have symptomatic hip dysplasia, a triradiate cartilage that is closed, and a concentric reduction of the femoral head on an AIR view. The contraindications to a Ganz osteotomy are moderate to severe osteoarthritis, an open triradiate cartilage, or a patient who does not have a concentric reduction of the femoral head. The advantages of this procedure over others is a single incision approach, osteotomies close to the acetabulum, allowing for outstanding correction ability, including medialization, maintenance of the pelvic ring integrity (therefore allowing for early activity without immobilization), minimal disruption of the pelvic outlet allowing for normal vaginal delivery, and that it provides the ability to look into the joint through a capsulotomy without concern for the acetabular blood supply [10].

Operative technique

The procedure is performed in the supine position on a radiolucent table. No elevation of either hip is used. Generally the author places an epidural catheter for intraoperative use to decrease blood loss and postoperative pain management. Although electromyographic monitoring has been performed with great success in identifying postoperative neurologic deficits [11], the author has found it to be too sensitive, yielding false-positive results. The author generally does not recommend using this technique during surgery.

The original description was to strip the muscles off the pelvis laterally and medially; however, this has changed [12–14]. The most common approach is through a modified Smith-Peterson approach in which the incision is done along the iliac crest down to the anterior superior iliac spine, and either extended more distally along the anterolateral proximal thigh or slightly medial to the anterior superior iliac spine [12]. The extension over the proximal thigh is used most often when it is necessary to look into the hip joint to address labral pathology. An anterior superior iliac spine osteotomy is created, and the attached tensor fascia lata and the sartorius are retracted medially. The inner pelvis is stripped of soft tissue and a blunt Hohmann retractor usually is placed into the sciatic notch. The anterior soft tissue dissection is done so that the iliocapsularis muscle is dissected sharply off the hip joint capsule and dissection is carried down on the medial aspect of the capsule, down to the ischium, to gain exposure for the first cut. The Ganz osteotome, which is angled at 50°, is used to begin the cut in the infracondyloid groove, just below the inferior acetabulum. The cut generally is visualized under fluoroscopy using the AP pelvis and false-profile images so that the depth of the cut can go to approximately 2.5 cm (Fig. 5A). The medial cortex is usually more challenging to osteotomize, and this is cut first, followed by the lateral cortex.

The second cut is made on the superior ramus beginning just medial to the iliopectineal eminence, angled at approximately 45° and is usually made with a straight osteotome (Fig. 5B). Care is taken to do subperiosteal dissection around the superior ramus to ensure that this does not prevent motion and Hohmann retractors are placed to protect the obturator neurovascular bundle during the osteotomy. To ensure that the osteotomy is complete, a large osteotome is levered within the osteotomy and movement should be visualized.

Attention next is turned to the third cut, which begins just below the anterior superior iliac spine. To make this osteotomy a small width of muscle is stripped off the lateral aspect of the pelvis. The cut is made with a saw and is directed straight toward the floor if the patient is positioned supine, and ends just lateral to the pelvic brim. The end point of this third cut initially is visualized with an osteotome placed at the end of this cut, using a false-profile fluoroscopy view to ensure that this is in the middle portion of the posterior column (Fig. 5C).

The fourth cut is made beginning just lateral to the pelvic brim at the end of the third cut and usually is made with a curved osteotome and travels along the posterior column. The osteotomy should bisect the distance between the posterior aspect of the posterior column and the posterior aspect of the acetabulum (Fig. 5D). A 0.5-inch osteotome usually is used and should be visualized directly as it travels down this posterior column. Several passes of the osteotome are necessary to traverse the posterior column so that as one completes this cut the acetabular fragment begins to move laterally. As this occurs, the osteotomy is propagated through the lateral aspect of the posterior column. A 6.0-mm diameter Schanz pin then is placed into the acetabular fragment once the osteotomy has been completed and is used to manipulate the fragment.

Manipulation of the acetabular fragment is the most challenging aspect of this operation, because the fragment is so mobile that it is possible to place the fragment anywhere in space. According to Ganz, however, there is only one position that achieves the optimum acetabular coverage (without over coverage) while medializing the joint to restore Shenton's line and maintaining normal acetabular version [15]. The tendency is to create retroversion as one rotates the fragment anteriorly (this is represented by the crossover sign on the AP radiograph in which the outline of the anterior wall ends more laterally than the posterior wall) [16]. Retroversion of the acetabulum may be present before surgery in patients who have hip dysplasia with a reported incidence of 16% to 33% [17,18]. The initial step to reorientation of the acetabulum is to ensure that the superior ramus cut is free and the superior ramus aspect of the acetabular fragment is moved proximal to the remaining superior ramus and then directed slightly posteriorly. Following this, the entire fragment then can be rotated predominantly anteriorly, which improves anterior and lateral coverage. It is often then necessary to hold onto the superior ramus aspect of the acetabular fragment with a bone reduction forceps, and using this in conjunction with the Schanz pin, the fragment then can be rotated appropriately.

Following completion of rotation, provisional fixation with K-wires is performed. At this point a fluoroscopy view or an AP pelvic radiograph is used to assess the position of the acetabular fragment. Several attempts at positioning the fragment are necessary to achieve optimal correction in all planes

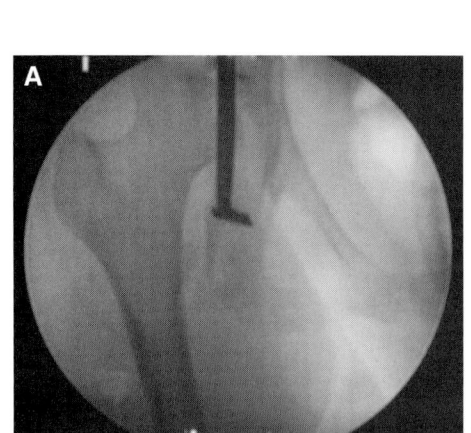
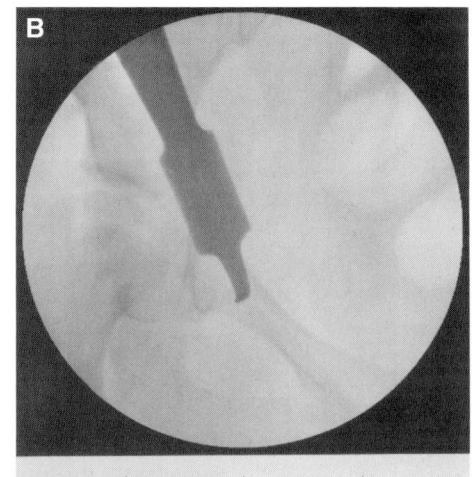
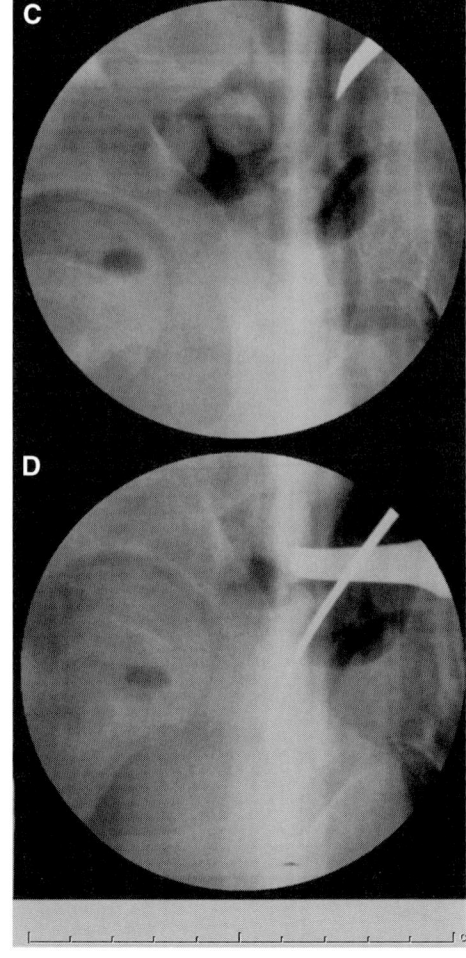

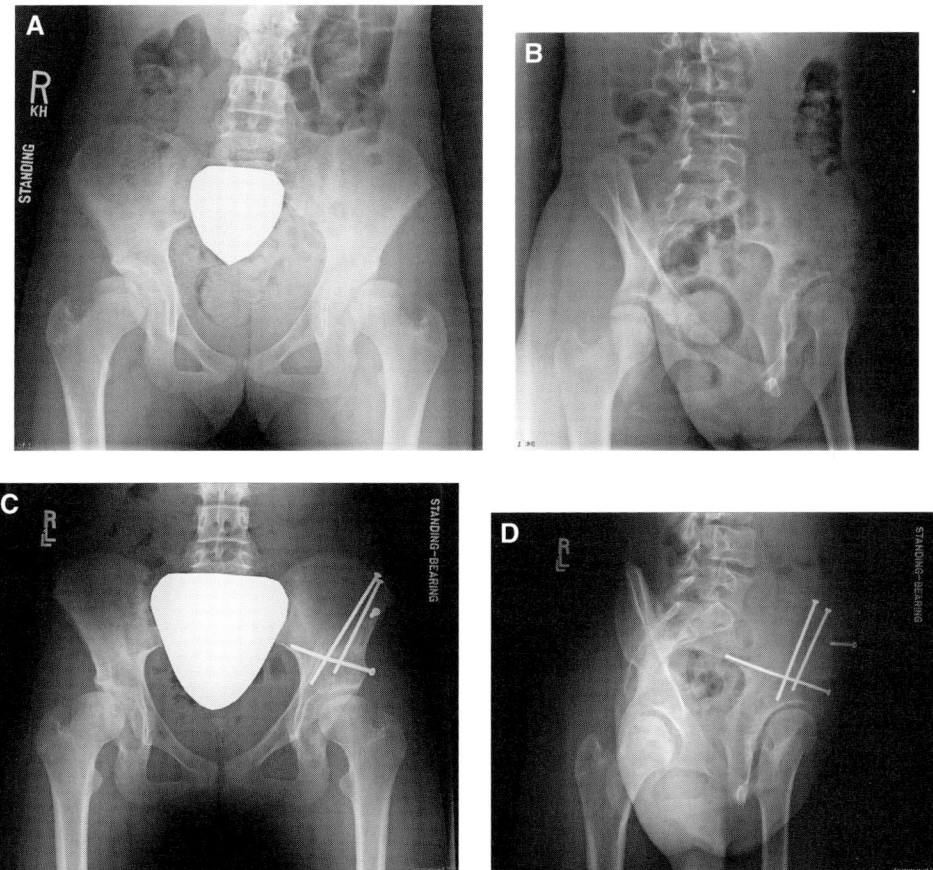

Fig. 6. A 14-year-old female with bilateral hip dysplasia who was symptomatic on the left. (*A*) The preoperative AP radiograph demonstrating bilateral hip dysplasia with an increase in the acetabular index of the weightbearing zone, an abnormal center edge angle without joint space narrowing or other signs of hip degeneration. (*B*) The false profile radiograph of the left hip demonstrating a loss of anterior hip coverage as evidence by a decrease in the ventral center edge angle. (*C*) An AP radiograph performed one year following the Ganz periacetabular osteotomy with restoration of the normal center edge angle, and a horizontal sourcil. Medialization of the hip joint center has also occurred with restoration of Shenton's line. Note that the acetabular version is normal with the anterior wall and posterior wall ending laterally together. (*D*) The 1-year postoperative false profile radiograph demonstrating excellent restoration of the anterior coverage.

while maintaining normal version (Fig. 6). Fixation of the acetabular fragment is varied, depending on the preference of the surgeon and the quality of the bone; however, three to four 3.5-mm or 4.5-mm screws provide excellent stability [19,20]. The screws generally are placed so that they are not close to the acetabular weightbearing surface to avoid interfering with potential future reconstruction options.

Patient outcomes

The results of the Ganz periacetabular osteotomy were first reported in 1988 by the developing surgeon for his initial 63 patients [3]. This report demonstrated excellent results in the short follow-up period and generated great enthusiasm for this procedure. The same patients (75 dysplastic hip joints) were re-

Fig. 5. Fluoroscopic images of the osteotomies performed. (*A*) The first cut being made using the Ganz osteotome visualized on a false-profile image. (*B*) The second cut is made on the superior ramus starting just medial to the iliopectineal eminence. (*C*) The third cut begins just distal to the anterior superior iliac spine and ends just lateral to the pelvic brim, which is a point that allows for the start of the fourth cut. (*D*) The fourth cut is made with a curved osteotome that travels down the central aspect of the posterior column.

evaluated at a minimum of 10 years [8]. Most patients were female and the average age was 29 years. Five of the 63 patients had an underlying neurologic condition, 2 patients had post-traumatic acetabular deficiency, and 2 additional patients had the diagnosis of proximal femoral focal deficiency. Previous surgery had been performed on 31% of the patients, and all patients underwent the procedure because of pain. Siebenrock and colleagues demonstrated that there was significant improvement in the lateral center edge angle, the anterior center edge angle, the acetabular index of the weightbearing zone, and medialization of the hip joint center. An unfavorable outcome was more common when there was a marked preoperative osteoarthritis, presence of a labral lesion, when surgery was performed on older patients, and on those patients who had less postoperative anterior femoral head coverage. They also reported on their complication rate, which was seen in the first 18 patients, without major complications in their subsequent procedures. The conclusion from this series is that patients overall do well, especially when the selection criteria are followed. Others have demonstrated similar results with the periacetabular osteotomy but with shorter follow-up [13,21–24].

Although the Ganz periacetabular osteotomy is used most commonly for otherwise normal patients who have hip dysplasia, its versatility allows for use in other conditions. MacDonald and colleagues reviewed 13 dysplastic hips in 11 adult patients who had underlying neurologic diagnoses and demonstrated overall good outcomes [25]. Seven hips were in patients who had flaccid paralysis, whereas six were in patients who had spasticity. The radiographic dysplasia improved, including the Tonnis angle ($33°-8°$), center edge angle ($-10°-25°$), and extrusion index (53%–15%). Pain improved in all 11 patients, with complete resolution in 7. The investigators concluded that this is a versatile osteotomy that can be used in the patient who has neurogenic underlying neurologic conditions. Katz and others demonstrated that the Ganz periacetabular osteotomy can be used effectively in patients who have Down syndrome [26]. The average age of their patients was 17 years, and they demonstrated improvement in the Tonnis acetabular angle, the lateral center edge angle, and the extrusion index. Two patients developed subluxation postoperatively, however, and required femoral osteotomies, whereas another patient developed a labral tear requiring arthroscopic debridement. In this difficult patient population, the author believes that the Ganz periacetabular osteotomy is a viable option to treat residual dysplasia.

Although the osteotomy is performed most easily in previously untreated patients who present with mild hip dysplasia, it also can be performed in patients who have had previous surgery and in those who have severe hip dysplasia. Mayo and colleagues analyzed 19 periacetabular osteotomies in 18 patients who had previous hip surgery and demonstrated similar radiographic improvement following the surgery when compared with a group of patients who had no previous surgery [27]. The clinical outcome was improved based on Harris hip scores and the Merle d'Aubigne index. Although most radiographic parameters (lateral center edge angle, anterior center edge angle, and acetabular index of the weightbearing zone) are improved, medialization can be difficult, and the surgical procedures are longer and have greater blood loss.

One of the advantages of the periacetabular osteotomy is that it is versatile and can be used in the patient who is mildly affected and in the severely dysplastic hip patient. Clohisy and colleagues reviewed 16 hips in 13 patients who were classified as having severe acetabular dysplasia by the Severin classification and who demonstrated significant improvement in all radiographic parameters analyzed. Clinical outcome was also improved, with increases in Harris hip scores from 73.4 points preoperatively to 91.3 points at the latest follow-up [28]. They concluded that the Ganz periacetabular osteotomy is an effective treatment for surgical correction of the severely dysplastic hip in the early follow-up period. They noted that proximal femoral varus osteotomy is often necessary in these patients to improve the overall relationship between the femoral head and the acetabulum. The author's experience has been that these patients also can be treated well with acetabular procedures, even in the face of previous surgical procedures (Fig. 7). The indication for varus osteotomy is changing, especially as surgeons become more adept at improving the horizontilization of the sourcil in these patients.

A total hip arthroplasty can be performed following a Ganz periacetabular osteotomy and may provide a better foundation to place the acetabular component. Parvizi and colleagues reviewed 41 patients who had total hip arthroplasty after the Ganz periacetabular osteotomy [29]. The total hip arthroplasty provided marked relief of symptoms. They noted some technical issues when performing the surgery including recognizing that the acetabulum was retroverted in 23 of the 41 patients studied. The anatomic landmarks should be evaluated carefully when placing the femoral and acetabular components.

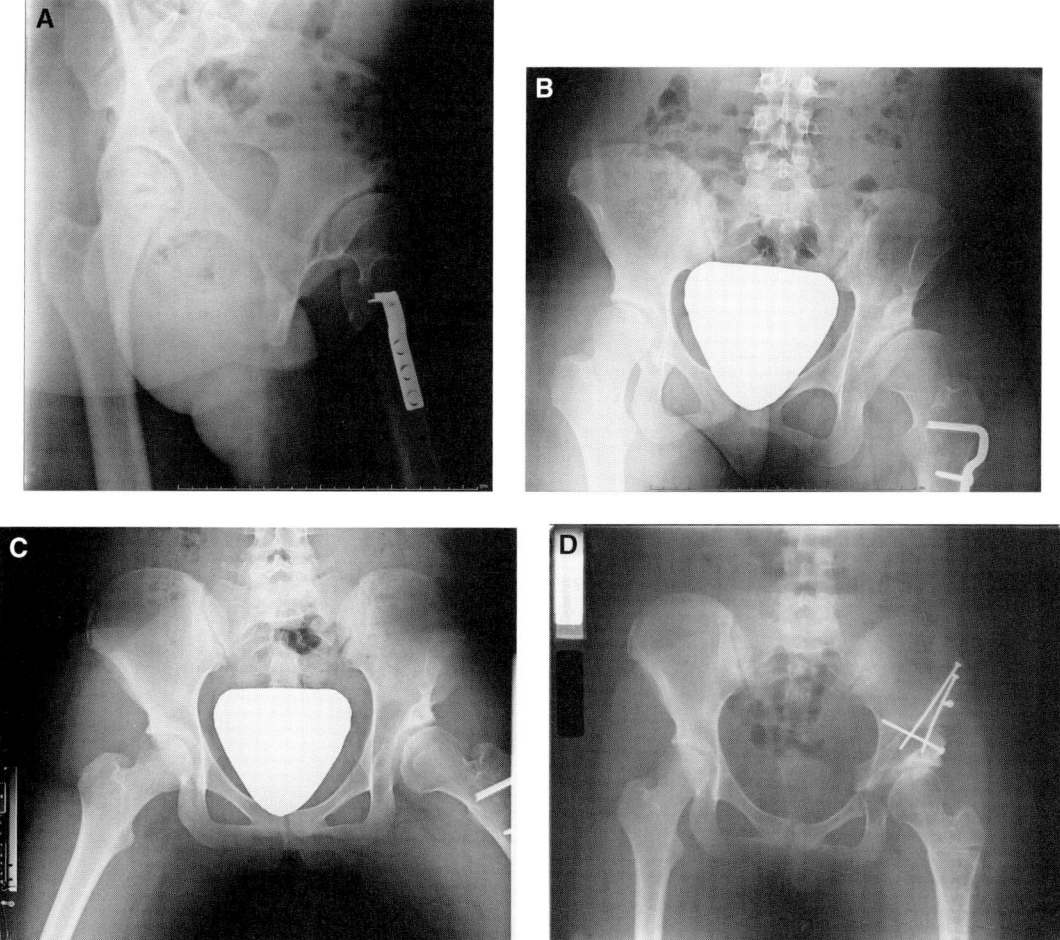

Fig. 7. A fairly typical radiographic appearance of a patient who had multiple previous surgeries for hip dysplasia performed at an outlying institution who presented with severe hip pain on the left. The preoperative radiographs demonstrate severe hip dysplasia on the AP and false-profile radiographs. The postoperative radiographs demonstrate significant improvement in the medialization of the acetabulum, horizontalization of the sourcil, and excellent femoral head coverage on the AP and false-profile radiographs.

Two of the concerns of surgeons performing this periacetabular osteotomy are the incidence of complications and the learning curve associated with this procedure. Davey and Santore demonstrated that there was a significant learning curve that is achieved by 35 cases in which their major complication rate dropped from 17% to 2.9% [30]. Ganz reviewed his experience with his periacetabular osteotomy and reported the incidence of complications from a group of 508 patients. The results demonstrated that the complications included intra-articular extension of the osteotomy (2.2%), insufficient or excessive correction (0.8%), subluxation of the femoral head (0.8%), transient femoral nerve palsy (0.6%), transient sciatic nerve palsy (1.0%), osteonecrosis of the acetabular fragment (0.6%), femoral head osteonecrosis (0.2%), posterior column discontinuity (1.2%), acetabular fragment migration (0.8%), and symptomatic proximal screw heads (3.0%). It is important for surgeons to read these studies and others [24] to understand the types of complications and methods to avoid them.

One of the advantages of the Ganz periacetabular osteotomy is that it does not result in disruption of the pelvic ring; this has been demonstrated nicely by Trousdale and colleagues when they showed no significant change in the osseous pelvis by magnetic resonance imaging pelvimetry [31]. The clinical sequela of this is that these predominantly young female patients can undergo vaginal deliveries [32]. They also demonstrated that patients had normal sexual activity, especially when acetabular retroversion was not seen, as this limited their range of motion and produced hip pain.

Summary

Hip dysplasia is common, seen more often in females, and presents with lateral or anterior hip pain. Patients may present with silent dysplasia, without having a previous history of dysplasia, or they may present with a long history including multiple surgeries. Hip dysplasia results in a suboptimal biomechanical hip situation that can lead to significant premature osteoarthritis. Reorientation of the acetabulum may prevent or certainly delay the onset of osteoarthritis. The Ganz periacetabular osteotomy had been well studied before its clinical application and was first reported in a series in 1998 by Ganz and colleagues. This reorientation procedure creates osteotomies close to the deformity and results in outstanding reorientation of the acetabulum in all planes. It is a technically challenging procedure; however, when well studied it can be performed safely and effectively with outstanding clinical outcomes.

References

[1] Cooperman DRW, Stulberg SD. Acetabular dysplasia in the adult. Clin Orthop Rel Res 1983;175:79–85.
[2] Stulberg SD, Harris WH. Acetabular dysplasia in the development of osteoarthritis of the hip. Paper presented at Proceedings of the Second Open Scientific Meeting of the Hip Society, St. Louis, MO, 1974.
[3] Ganz R, Klaue K, Vinh TS, et al. A new periacetabular osteotomy for the treatment of hip dysplasias. Technique and preliminary results. Clin Orthop 1988;232: 26–36.
[4] Klaue K, Durnin CW, Ganz R. The acetabular rim syndrome. A clinical presentation of dysplasia of the hip. J Bone Joint Surg [Br] 1991;73(3):423–9.
[5] Horii M, Kubo T, Inoue S, et al. Coverage of the femoral head by the acetabular labrum in dysplastic hips: quantitative analysis with radial MR imaging. Acta Orthop Scand 2003;74(3):287–92.
[6] Leunig M, Werlen S, Ungersböck A, et al. Evaluation of the acetabular labrum by MR arthrography. J Bone Joint Surg [Br] 1997;79(2):230–4.
[7] Leunig M, Podeszwa D, Beck M, et al. Magnetic resonance arthrography of labral disorders in hips with dysplasia and impingement. Clin Orthop 2004; 418:74–80.
[8] Siebenrock KA, Schöll E, Lottenbach M, et al. Bernese periacetabular osteotomy. Clin Orthop Rel Res 1999; 363:9–20.
[9] Kim Y-J, Jaramillo D, Millis MB, et al. Assessment of early osteoarthritis in hip dysplasia with delayed gadolinium-enhanced magnetic resonance imaging of cartilage. J Bone Joint Surg [Am] 2003;85-A(10): 1987–92.
[10] Beck M, Leunig M, Ellis T, et al. The acetabular blood supply: implications for periacetabular osteotomies. Surgical and radiologic anatomy. SRA 2003;25(5–6): 361–7.
[11] Pring ME, Trousdale RT, Cabanela ME, et al. Intraoperative electromyographic monitoring during periacetabular osteotomy. Clin Orthop Rel Res 2002;400: 158–64.
[12] Murphy SB, Millis MB. Periacetabular osteotomy without abductor dissection using direct anterior exposure. Clin Orthop Rel Res 1999;364:92–8.
[13] Matta JM, Stover MD, Siebenrock K. Periacetabular osteotomy through the Smith-Petersen approach. Clin Orthop Rel Res 1999;363:21–32.
[14] Hussell JG, Mast JW, Mayo KA, et al. A comparison of different surgical approaches for the periacetabular osteotomy. Clin Orthop Rel Res 1999;363:64–72.
[15] Hussell JG, Rodriguez JA, Ganz R. Technical complications of the Bernese periacetabular osteotomy. Clin Orthop Rel Res 1999;363:81–92.
[16] Ganz R, Parvizi J, Beck M, et al. Femoroacetabular impingement: a cause for osteoarthritis of the hip. Clin Orthop Rel Res 2003;417:112–20.
[17] Li PLS, Ganz R. Morphologic features of congenital acetabular dysplasia: one in six is retroverted. Clin Orthop Rel Res 2003;416:245–53.
[18] Mast JW, Brunner RL, Zebrack J. Recognizing acetabular version in the radiographic presentation of hip dysplasia. Clin Orthop Rel Res 2004;418:48–53.
[19] Yassir W, Mahar A, Aminian A, et al. A comparison of the fixation stability of multiple screw constructs for two types of pelvic osteotomies. J Pediatr Orthop 2005;25(1):14–7.
[20] Babis GC, Trousdale RT, Jenkyn TR, et al. Comparison of two methods of screw fixation in periacetabular osteotomy. Clin Orthop Rel Res 2002;403:221–7.
[21] Murphy SB, Millis MB, Hall JE. Surgical correction of acetabular dysplasia in the adult. A Boston experience. Clin Orthop Rel Res 1999;363:38–44.
[22] Pogliacomi F, Stark A, Wallensten R. Periacetabular osteotomy. Good pain relief in symptomatic hip dysplasia, 32 patients followed for 4 years. Acta Orthop Scand 2005;76(1):67–74.
[23] Pogliacomi F, Stark A, Vaienti E, et al. Periacetabular osteotomy of the hip: the ilioinguinal approach. Acta bio-medica de L'Ateneo parmense: organo della Società di medicina e scienze naturali di Parma. ACTA Biomed Ateneo Parmense 2003;74(1):38–46.

[24] Trousdale RT, Cabanela ME. Lessons learned after more than 250 periacetabular osteotomies. Acta Orthop Scand 2003;74(2):119–26.
[25] McDonald GA. Pelvic disruptions in children. Clin Orthop 1980;151:130–4.
[26] Katz DA, Kim Y-J, Millis MB. Periacetabular osteotomy in patients with Down's syndrome. J Bone Joint Surg [Br] 2005;87(4):544–7.
[27] Mayo KA, Trumble SJ, Mast JW. Results of periacetabular osteotomy in patients with previous surgery for hip dysplasia. Clin Orthop Rel Res 1999;363:73–80.
[28] Clohisy JC, Barrett SE, Gordon JE, et al. Periacetabular osteotomy for the treatment of severe acetabular dysplasia. J Bone Joint Surg [Am] 2005;87(2):254–9.
[29] Parvizi J, Burmeister H, Ganz R. Previous Bernese periacetabular osteotomy does not compromise the results of total hip arthroplasty. Clin Orthop Rel Res 2004;423:118–22.
[30] Davey JP, Santore RF. Complications of periacetabular osteotomy. Clin Orthop Rel Res 1999;363:33–7.
[31] Trousdale RT, Cabanela ME, Berry DJ, et al. Magnetic resonance imaging pelvimetry before and after a periacetabular osteotomy. J Bone Joint Surg [Am] 2002;84-A(4):552–6.
[32] Valenzuela RG, Cabanela ME, Trousdale RT. Sexual activity, pregnancy, and childbirth after periacetabular osteotomy. Clin Orthop Rel Res 2004;418:146–52.

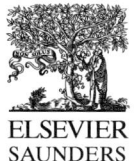

Operative Reconstruction for Septic Arthritis of the Hip

In Ho Choi, MD*, Won Joon Yoo, MD, Tae-Joon Cho, MD, Chin Youb Chung, MD

Department of Orthopedic Surgery, Seoul National University Hospital, 28 Yongon-dong, Chongno-gu, Seoul 110–744, Korea

The long-term effects of initial treatment for infantile septic arthritis of the hip may differ and depend on patient age, the infecting organism, and the timing and adequacy of surgical and pharmacologic treatment [1–5]. Sequelae are diverse and include necrosis of the cartilage, ischemic necrosis of the femoral head, premature closure of the triradiate cartilage, acetabular dysplasia, premature or asymmetric closure of the proximal femoral physis, subluxation, dislocation, pseudarthrosis of the femoral neck, greater trochanteric overriding, and complete destruction of the femoral head and neck [1,2,6–8]. When severe destruction of the proximal femur with loss of physeal growth occurs, functional disabilities are enormous in affected children. Such children often present with clinical problems such as pain, limp, and hip instability, or even emotional disturbances.

When only a remnant of the femoral head and neck is present, maintaining a stable reduction is difficult, and if instability and dislocation persist, one is left with the decision to accept the deformity or to attempt reconstruction of a femoral–pelvic articulation [9]. Continued observation results in proximal iliac dislocation with a marked abductor lurch, a telescoping limp, and leg-length inequality [7,10]. Although these patients may do well for several years [2,6,11], they are at risk for degenerative changes in the lumbosacral spine and hip. Moreover, surgical treatment of the hip is difficult because of secondary loss of bone stock [9]. The available means of reconstructive procedures for the treatment of severe sequelae are limited and in general have not yielded satisfactory long-term results [1,2,6,9,11]. Few long-term follow-up studies have been reported in the literature on the management of residual deformities, and available reports include only small numbers of patients who have severe sequelae.

Appropriate and timely reconstructive operations would benefit hip growth and development by providing the best possible hip joint mechanics at skeletal maturity. Moreover, some of the aforementioned complications caused by observation alone can be avoided. Any surgical treatment for severe sequelae must be regarded as a measure that temporarily improves clinical function, however, and delays the more definitive procedures that are reserved for adult patients [1]. This article summarizes the surgical modalities currently available to reduce and stabilize a damaged femoral head and neck and to reconstruct femoral–acetabular articulation.

Radiographic classifications of late sequelae

Radiologic classification of residual femoral deformities was developed to classify residual deformities based on the nature and extent of injury and radiographic appearance at final follow-up or maturity, and each was further divided into two subgroups (Fig. 1) [1].

Type I

In these hips, the growth of the proximal femoral ossification center results in an almost normal hip

No benefits in any form have been received or will be received from any commercial party related directly or indirectly to the subject of this article.
* Corresponding author.
E-mail address: inhoc@snu.ac.kr (I.H. Choi).

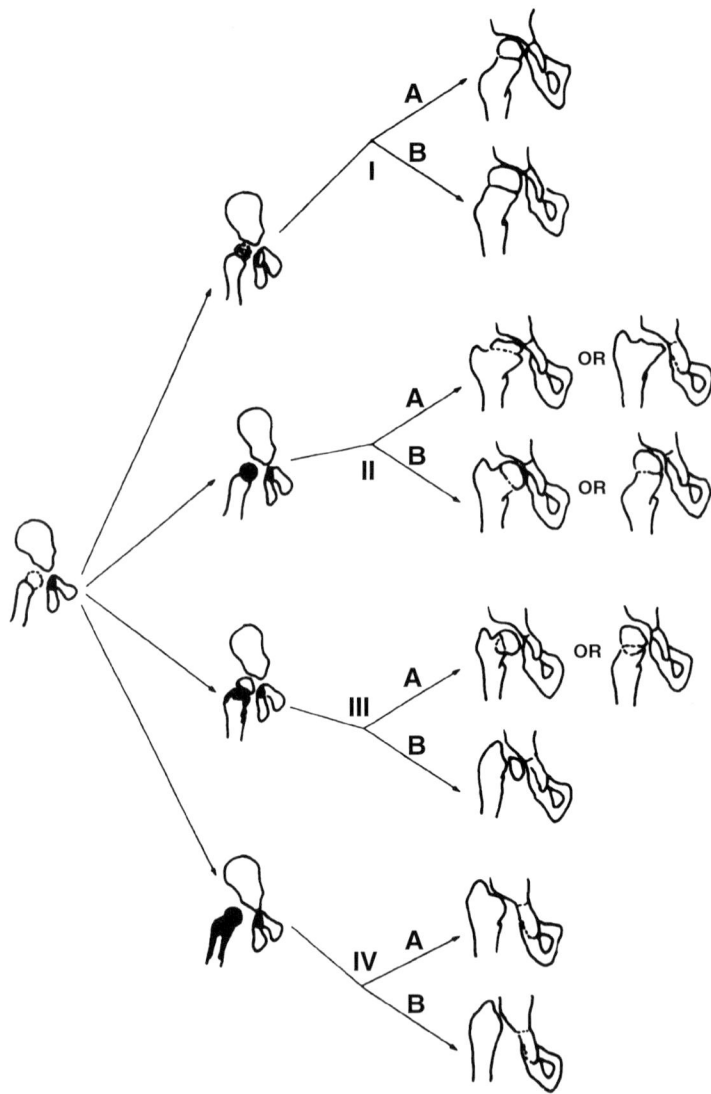

Fig. 1. Classification of sequelae. Type I, no residual deformity (type IA) or mild coxa magna (type IB). Type II, coxa breva with a deformed head (type IIA) or progressive coxa vara or valga caused by asymmetric, premature physeal closure (type IIB). Type III, slipping at the femoral neck resulting in coxa vara or valga with severe anteversion or retroversion (type IIIA) or pseudarthrosis of the femoral neck (type IIIB). Type IV, destruction of the femoral head and neck with a small remnant of the neck (type IVA) or complete loss of the femoral head and neck and no articulation of the hip (type IVB). (*From* Choi IH, Pizzutillo PD, Bowen JR, et al. Sequelae and reconstruction after septic arthritis of the hip in infants. J Bone Joint Surg 1990;72A(8):1150–65; with permission.)

(type IA) or in mild coxa magna (type IB). For type I deformities, delay of ossification, mottling, or fragmentation of the proximal femoral ossific nucleus is followed by rapid and complete re-ossification, the proximal femoral physis remains viable with little or no shortening of the femoral neck, and acetabular development is adequate.

Type II

The epiphysis, physis, and metaphysis are involved, with resulting coxa breva (type IIA) or progressive coxa vara or coxa valgus (type IIB). These hips usually have radiographic evidence of delayed ossification, flattening and irregularity of the femoral head, and coxa magna. The femoral neck is short and wide, and there is relative overgrowth of the greater trochanter because of premature closure of the capital physis. When there is early symmetric closure of the proximal femoral physis (type IIA), coxa breva with overriding of the trochanter develops, which is associated with a resultant limp and considerable limb-length discrepancy. When premature physeal closure is asymmetric and incomplete, the femoral neck progressively grows into varus or valgus alignment with secondary acetabular dysplasia.

Type III

In these hips, the deformity is secondary to injury of the femoral neck and results in angular deformity with severe anteversion or retroversion (type IIIA) or in pseudarthrosis (type IIIB). This deformity is reported infrequently and may be secondary to osteomyelitis of the femoral neck. Hips that have type-IIIA sequelae have severe coxa vara or coxa valga in association with extreme anteversion or retroversion, whereas those with type-IIIB sequelae have pseudarthrosis of the femoral neck with complete epiphyseal slipping. These changes result in an altered acetabular development, limb-length discrepancy, and relative trochanteric overgrowth.

Type IV

In type IV, the most severe type, compromise of the femoral head and neck results in an unstable hip with a persistent remnant of the femoral neck (type IVA) or in complete loss of the femoral head and neck with no vestige of an articulation (type IVB). These hips have the most unpredictable radiographic findings at follow up, with severe limb-length discrepancy, acetabular dysplasia, premature closure of the triradiate cartilage, and marked proximal migration of the femur, with or without the formation of a false acetabulum.

The classification system of Hunka [8] does not seem to have a subtype equivalent to the Choi type IIIA, though Hunka types IV and V deformities are equivalent to Choi types IVA and IVB.

Algorithmic treatment strategy for hip reconstruction

Once the anatomy of a hip is defined after initial treatment, including conservative treatment, a surgical

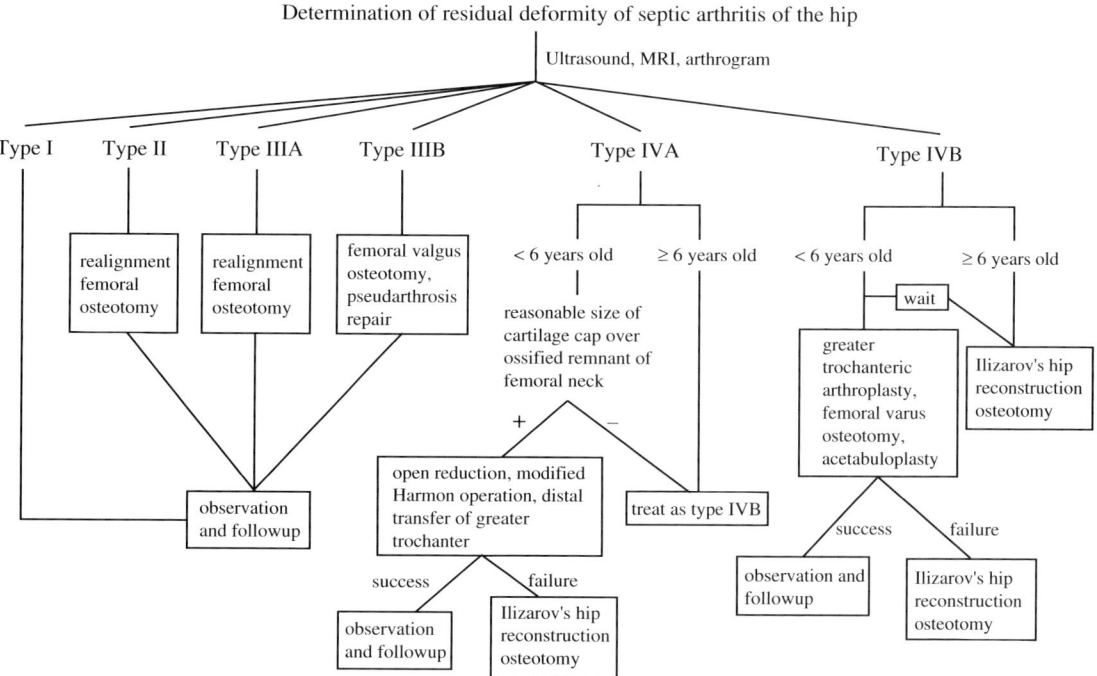

Fig. 2. The devised algorithmic protocol for the treatment of sequelae of infantile septic arthritis of the hip. (*From* Choi IH, Shin YW, Chung CY, et al. Surgical treatment of the severe sequelae of infantile septic arthritis of the hip. Clin Orthop Relat Res 2005;434:108; with permission.)

treatment can be formulated. Modern imaging tools, including MRI, ultrasonography, and arthrography are helpful at determining early how much of the femoral head and neck is present, whether it is located, subluxated, or dislocated, and whether there is any associated damage on the acetabulum. The authors recently proposed an algorithmic treatment protocol for the different types of sequelae (Fig. 2) [12]. This protocol is based on the authors' experiences of 147 hips in 144 patients treated for septic hip sequelae during 1980 and 2002 at the authors' institution and on literature review. Forty-five hips in 43 patients had high-grade sequelae, ie, Choi types III and IV.

If the femoral head seems normal and is located, as seen in hips of types IA and IB, no reconstructive operation is needed because outcomes are generally good. Hips with type II deformity, however, need an operation to prevent subluxation; the goals of the operation include improved acetabular coverage, improved abductor efficiency by epiphysiodesis or transfer of the greater trochanter, and equalization of limb-length inequality, primarily by epiphysiodesis of the contralateral limb. If there is substantial coxa brevis, Wagner-type neck-lengthening [13] would be beneficial for proximal femur reconstruction to reduce pain and provide improved hip function and bone stock for any future definitive replacement arthroplasty. Similarly, in hips with type IIIA sequelae with any severe coxa vara or valga with torsional malalignment, early femoral corrective osteotomy is efficacious at restoring a normal femoral neck-shaft angle and reorienting the growth plate in a more favorable direction with respect to biomechanical stresses. As opposed to type IIIA, type IIIB sequelae are difficult to treat, particularly when associated with a mobile nonunion of the femoral neck. Every effort should be made to achieve osteosynthesis of the neck by valgus osteotomy and pseudarthrosis repair with bone grafting. For type IVA in patients younger than 6 years of age with a reasonable size unossified cartilage cap over the neck remnant, the repositioning of the femoral remnant into the acetabular socket by open reduction can be facilitated using the authors' modification of the Harmon operation [12,14]. This procedure provides a neck-lengthening effect by making an incomplete spring osteotomy at the base of the femoral remnant adjoining the greater trochanter and filling the resulting opening wedged gap with a block of cartilage graft taken from the iliac apophysis. Nonetheless, secondary procedures usually are needed to improve acetabular coverage and abductor efficiency by epiphysiodesis or transfer of the greater trochanter and to equalize limb-length discrepancy, usually by lengthening the affected limb with or without epiphysiodesis of the contralateral limb. If this fails, an Ilizarov pelvic support osteotomy can be substituted. Children older than 6 years can be treated as type IVB. If a child has type IVB and is younger than 6 years, trochanter arthroplasty with acetabuloplasty can be performed selectively. Ilizarov hip reconstruction osteotomy is preferred in older patients who have type IVB or type IVA sequelae with unsuccessful previous reconstructive surgery or who present late with severe abductor lurch and considerable limb-length discrepancy.

Greater trochanteric arthroplasty

Trochanteric arthroplasty as described originally by Colonna [15] was popularized by Westin [16] and others [10,17,18]. The underlying concept is based on the following two aspects: (1) the greater trochanter is viable and therefore retains its growth potential, and (2) when the hyaline cartilage covering the trochanter is placed inside the influence of the acetabulum, the trochanter tends to assume a globular shape, similar to a femoral head [19]. The detached abductor muscles must be transferred downward to provide hip stability and some degree of abductor function. The subsequent progressive subluxation encountered in most patients, however, necessitates additional procedures, such as femoral osteotomy, pelvic osteotomy, and acetabuloplasty, to maintain coverage and containment (Fig. 3). Trochanteric arthroplasty has many problems and limitations associated with the uniqueness of the technique for the reconstruction of femoral–pelvic articulation [1,9,10,17–19]: (1) avascularity of the proximal segment after femoral varus osteotomy, (2) difficulty in osteosynthesis at the varus osteotomy site, (3) gradual straightening of proximal femur caused by remodeling at the osteotomy site, (4) abductor weakness, (5) stiffness, (6) degenerative arthritis, and (7) difficulty converting to total hip arthroplasty in adulthood. Of these, preoperative abductor weakness and stiffness are the two most important key factors that determine procedure success or failure.

Pelvic support osteotomy

The Ilizarov hip reconstruction is a combination of proximal pelvic support osteotomy for valgus angulation and extension and a distal femoral osteotomy to correct limb-length discrepancy by femoral lengthening and extremity realignment [20–26].

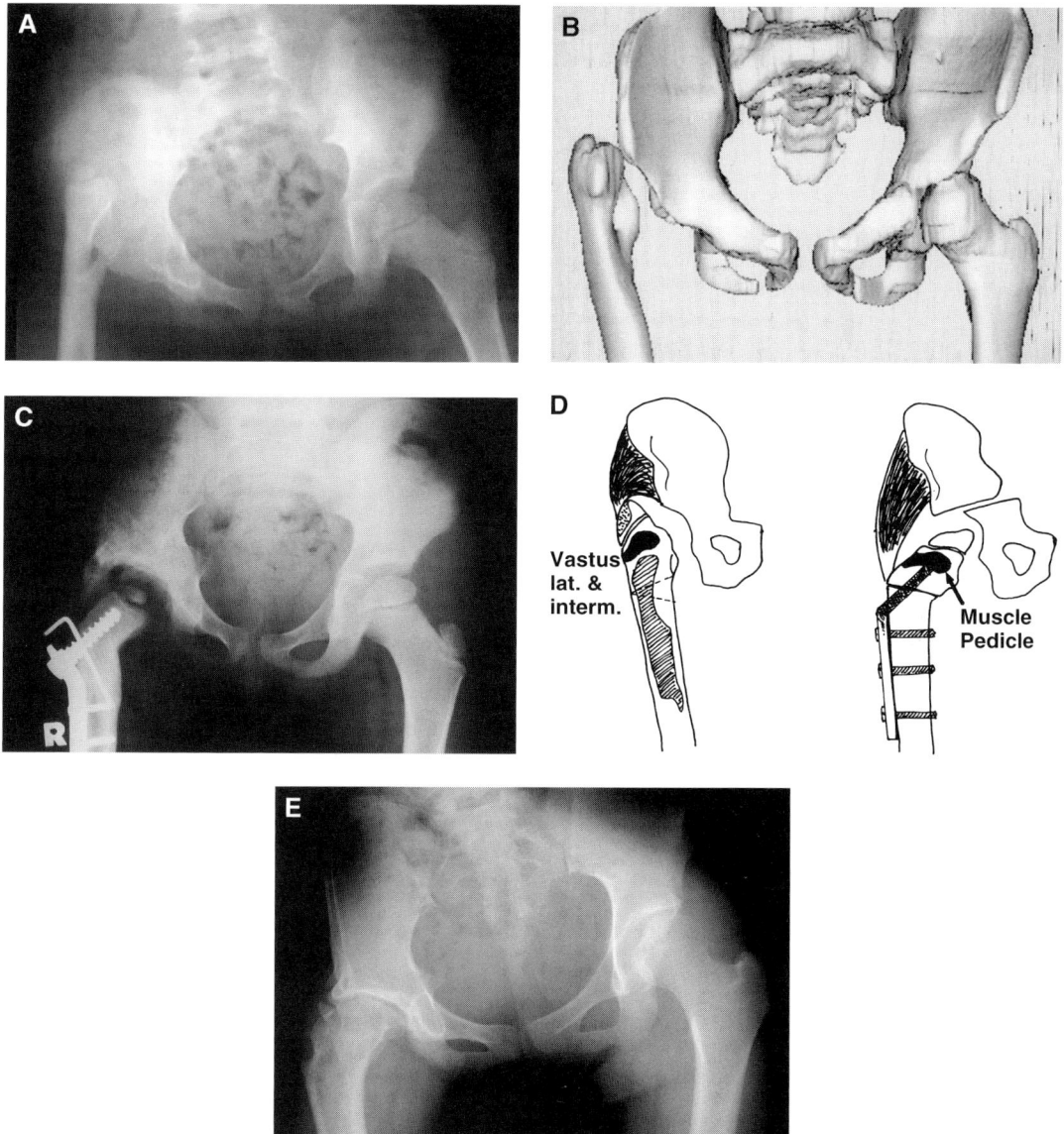

Fig. 3. Trochanteric arthroplasty in a girl. (A) A 5-year-old girl with Choi type IVB sequelae in the right hip with resultant severe pelvic obliquity. (B) A 3-D computed tomography image of the right hip showing complete loss of the femoral head and neck and premature closure of triradiate cartilage. (C) A radiograph taken 6 months after trochanteric arthroplasty with adjunctive femoral varus osteotomy and Chiari osteotomy. (D) A schematic drawing depicting the authors' modification of muscle-pedicled trochanteric arthroplasty. The origin of the vastus lateralis and intermedius was not detached during dissection in an attempt to preserve vascularity in the proximal fragment after femoral osteotomy. (E) A radiograph taken at 14 years of age showing a well-remodeled greater trochanter that had assumed a globular shape similar to that of a femoral head.

To better understand the evolution of Ilizarov hip reconstruction osteotomy, it may be useful to describe briefly the historical proximal femoral osteotomies used to treat old neglected dislocations of the hip. An angulated subtrochanteric osteotomy of the femur to support the acetabulum and stabilize the hip has been proposed by many previous investigators [27–29]. The osteotomies described by these investigators were based on the concept of surgically shifting the femur closer to the center of gravity so that the body weight is transferred more directly along the axis of the femoral shaft. The Lorenz bifurcation osteotomy [27], in which the proximal end of the distal segment is displaced into the acetabulum with the capsule serving as an interposed membrane, was designed to support the pelvis on the osteotomized proximal part of the femur. The pelvic-support osteotomy of Schanz [28] was designed to produce stability in a dislocated hip by valgus angulation osteotomy, whereby the lesser trochanter usually was placed into the acetabulum, leaving the dislocation unreduced. Two primary goals are achieved by these types of reconstructions, although the hip joint is not approached directly, ie, stability enhancement and displacement of the center of gravity medially. The operations often reduce lurch and increase the functional length of a limb by abducting the distal fragment. Later, Milch expanded the concept and popularized pelvic support osteotomy in the United States [30,31]. He advocated subtrochanteric valgus osteotomy to improve hip mechanics but cautioned against excessive valgus. Two opposed goals are implicit in the aforementioned anecdotal procedures, for although excessive valgus angulation improves hip stability by increasing the mechanical efficiency of the abductor muscles, it also causes valgus malalignment of the knee and abutment of the proximal part of the femur against the pelvis, which may cause impingement pain when a patient attempts to adduct the lower extremity to a neutral position. The compromise is less abduction, which is not favored from the hip stability viewpoint, and the elimination of Trendelenburg gait. Lower limb-length discrepancy is not addressed by conventional pelvic support osteotomy [26].

Ilizarov hip reconstruction osteotomy is unique because it simultaneously addresses hip instability and the limb-length discrepancy in one operation [20–26]. By combining acute valgus angular osteotomy in the proximal femur and gradual femoral lengthening in the distal femur, both problems can be treated simultaneously and the need for multiple surgical procedures avoided. Proximal femoral osteotomy places the proximal femur in maximum adduction in relation to the pelvis. The effect of this osteotomy is not only to place the femur under the pelvis, and as a result to support the pelvis and to resolve Trendelenburg limp, because the pelvis cannot drop. Elimination of hip adduction requires overcorrection of 15° to 20° during valgus osteotomy, according to previous experience [24,26] (Fig. 4). Furthermore, Ilizarov emphasized extension of proximal femoral osteotomy to correct fixed flexion deformity of the hip and to permit locking of the hip joint. The biomechanics of hips are improved substantially by these corrections. Valgus alignment of the proximal part of the femur repositions the greater trochanter and the abductor muscle insertion laterally and distally. Lateralization increases the length of the abductor lever arm, and the distal shift tensions previously redundant gluteal muscles. The valgus alignment also creates a fulcrum at the medial end of the pelvic support. The net effect is a marked improvement in the function of the hip abductor mechanism. Moreover, extension of the osteotomy contributes to this by stabilizing the hip in the sagittal plane during single-limb stance. A second osteotomy in the distal metaphyseal or metaphyseal–diaphyseal area of the femur is used to lengthen the limb by distraction osteogenesis and to restore the normal mechanical axis [20–26].

A good understanding of the natural history of the sequelae of infantile septic arthritis of the hip is essential for the development of an effective treatment plan to ensure the best possible results in adulthood [1]. Recommended primary and secondary methods of treatment are as varied as the types of deformities, but unfortunately no definite primary treatment for severely damaged hips is capable of withstanding the forces imposed by these otherwise normal children or by the long-term demands of their activities [1]. For this reason, the effectiveness of late operative procedures at reducing or stabilizing a damaged femoral head into the acetabulum remain controversial, particularly when only a remnant of the femoral head neck is present.

Type IV hips are the most difficult to treat and have not provided satisfactory long-term results [1,2,6,8,12]. In young children in whom the femoral head and neck have been destroyed, as in type IVA sequelae, a new femoral neck can be fashioned to articulate with the acetabulum by using the L'Episcopo [32] or Harmon [14] reconstructions. When a reasonably sized unossified cartilaginous cap remains as a continuation of the femoral neck remnant, open reduction can be attempted. The repositioning of the femoral remnant into the acetabular socket can be facilitated using the aforementioned investigators' modification of the Harmon operation [12]. If a child is older, gradual lengthening of the remnant femoral neck using the Ilizarov technique [33] may be indicated. Nonetheless, the authors believe that open reduction at more than 6 years of age is not likely to be beneficial because of a high risk for stiffness and pain. The authors thus recommend that these hips should be treated in the same manner as hips with type IVB sequelae.

Various treatment modalities have been developed to reconstruct a femoral–pelvic articulation in hips

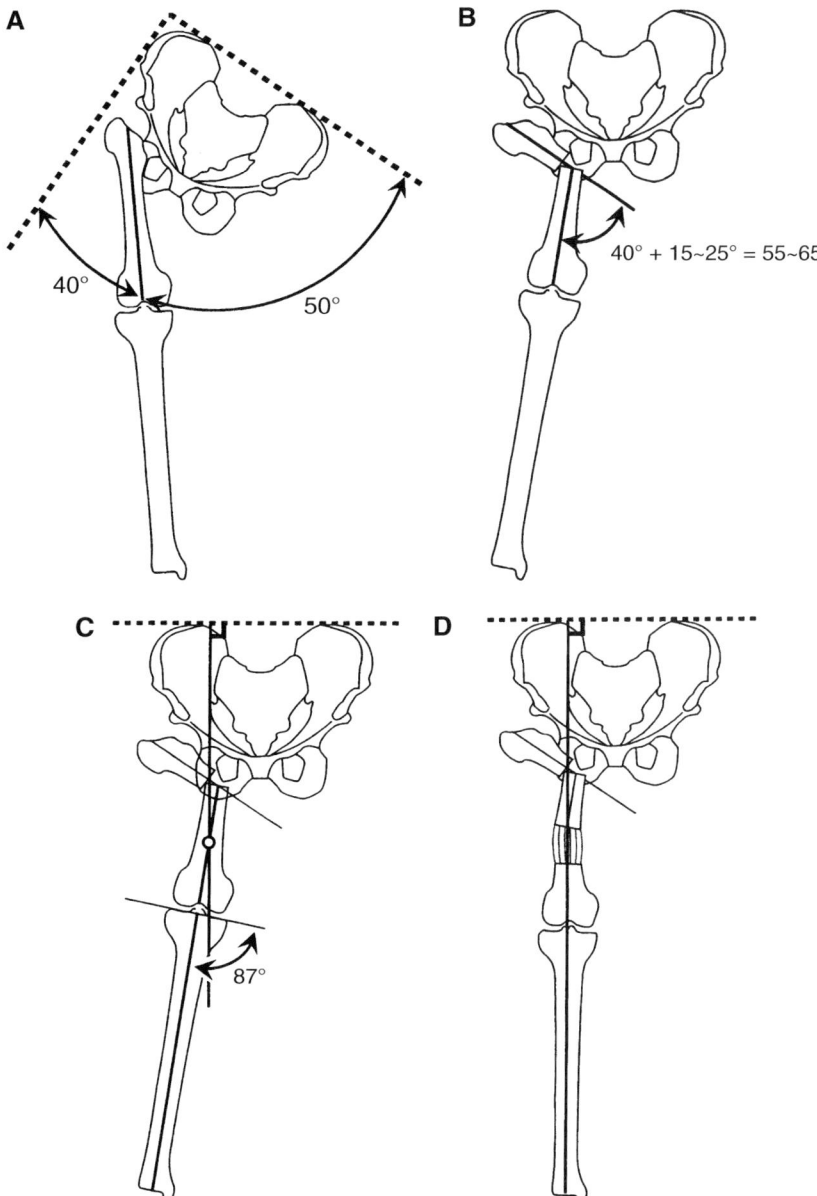

Fig. 4. Schematic diagrams of surgical planning. (*A*) Schematic representation of a single-limb–stance radiograph showing 40° of adduction and a Trendelenburg sign. Femoral adduction relative to a horizontal pelvic line represents the pelvic drop associated with the Trendelenburg sign. (*B*) Calculation of the desired angle of proximal osteotomy. A total of 15° to 25° is added to the amount of adduction as shown in Fig. 4*A*. (*C*) Determination of distal osteotomy level and the degree of varus correction required according to the intersection between the proximal and distal mechanical axis lines. The proximal mechanical axis is a line perpendicular to the horizontal line of the pelvis that passes through the proximal femoral osteotomy site. The distal mechanical axis line is a line from the center of the ankle that passes through the center of the knee. (*D*) Schematic diagram of a radiograph made at the end of distraction showing the proximal and the distal osteotomy. (*From* Paley D. Principles of deformity correction. New York: Springer; 2002. p. 689–90; with permission.)

with type IVB sequelae, eg, greater trochanteric arthroplasty [9,10,15–18] with adjunctive or secondary procedures, femoral head reconstruction with vascularized iliac crest grafting [34], Ilizarov hip reconstruction osteotomy [20–26], arthrodesis, and even observation without surgical intervention [2,4,11]. If a patient presents with a painful stiff hip, arthrodesis, although rare, may be indicated. Cheng and colleagues [34] used a technique involving the placement of a pedicled vascularized iliac crest graft to replace a destroyed femoral head and neck as an alternative to trochanteric arthroplasty. They reviewed their experience of eight hips in seven children with Choi type-IVB sequelae. Excellent graft incorporation was observed in three hips. The long-term evolution of this femoral head and neck reconstruction has yet to be determined, however, and the authors have experienced two cases of unsatisfactory results following vascularized iliac crest grafting caused by osteosynthesis failure, partial graft resorption, and stiffness [12].

Although some investigators have reported satisfactory results for the reconstruction of femoral–pelvic articulation by trochanteric arthroplasty [9,10,15,16], most surgeons with experience believe that trochanteric arthroplasty is a technically demanding procedure and that outcomes are highly unpredictable. According to the authors' retrospective study [12], satisfactory results were obtained in only 5 of 10 hips treated by trochanteric arthroplasty, and this occurred despite impressive remodeling of the transferred greater trochanter, which resembled a femoral head in most hips. Moreover, these results were found to be correlated with age at operation. In the study, all three patients who underwent trochanteric arthroplasty at an age older than 6 years demonstrated unsatisfactory results, whereas only two of seven patients who underwent trochanteric arthroplasty at less than 6 years of age had unsatisfactory results. This observation may support the opinion that a patient should be old enough to follow physical therapy instructions and young enough to allow remodeling of the transferred greater trochanter. Patients who exhibited unsatisfactory results showed stiffness despite multiple operations, a marked pelvic tilt, and a positive Trendelenburg sign caused by weak abductor power. These findings may indicate problems and difficulties when total hip replacement arthroplasty is undertaken in the future.

In contrast, the authors found that all five hips treated by Ilizarov hip reconstruction osteotomy were satisfactory regarding hip stability and range of motion and that these patients were free of pain [12]. Ilizarov hip reconstruction was found to be highly effective at eliminating or reducing Trendelenburg gait and at equalizing lower limb-length. The authors therefore currently prefer Ilizarov hip reconstruction osteotomy for the management of type IVB and IVA sequelae that have failed previous reconstructive surgery or that have presented late with severe abductor lurch and considerable limb-length discrepancy.

Some controversy exists concerning the optimal level required for pelvic support osteotomy and optimal age at operation regarding loss of valgus angulation by remodeling. Pelvic support can be achieved at the acetabular level by inserting the lesser trochanter into the acetabulum. The authors agree with Paley [22,26], however, that pelvic support at the subacetabular level resulting in a longer proximal segment provides better biomechanical advantages than that achieved at the acetabular level. This is attributed to a more medial fulcrum location because of a lower proximal osteotomy level. Medialization of the fulcrum decreases the abductor force needed to balance the weight of the body in single-limb stance. Moreover, the inferior aspect of the pelvis (subacetabular), near the ischial tuberosity, provides an optimal location for a soft-tissue interpositional weightbearing surface without direct abutment between the apex of a proximal femoral osteotomy and the pelvis.

Bone remodeling and subsequent gradual loss of valgus angulation remain important considerations in proximal femoral osteotomy (Fig. 5) [35–37]. In patients aged 9 to 17 years, loss of correction was reported to vary between 3° and 13° [20,31]; moreover, if the procedure is performed during earlier childhood, the femur almost completely straightens by the end of skeletal growth. Rozbruch and colleagues [26] found that in two patients who underwent proximal femoral osteotomy just distal to the level of the lesser trochanter (a high osteotomy) at a young age, osteotomy sites were completely remodeled and showed no evidence of pelvic support within 1 or 2 years postoperatively. The authors also have experienced a tendency toward femur straightening at the level of proximal osteotomy in growing children. When performing Ilizarov hip reconstruction osteotomy before adolescence, the authors therefore determine total valgus correction angle based on the single-leg stance drop angle relative to the horizontal line of the pelvis and add 25° of overcorrection [22,26] (see Fig. 4). In view of the gradual loss of valgus angulation by remodeling at the proximal osteotomy site in younger patients, some previous investigators [23,26] insisted that Ilizarov hip reconstruction is most suitable for skeletally mature ado-

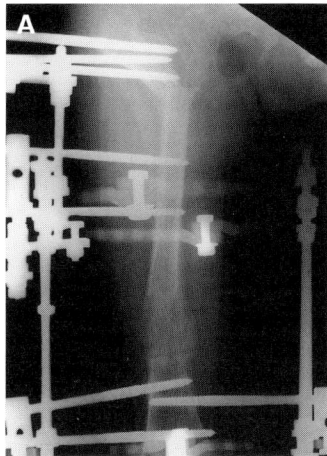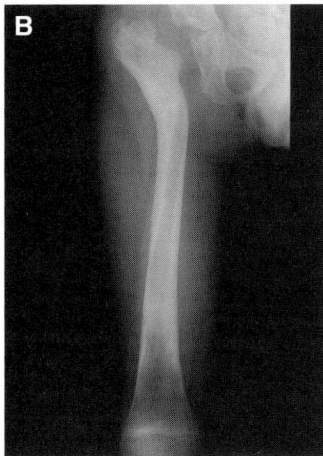

Fig. 5. (*A*) An anteroposterior radiograph of the right femur in a 6-year-old boy who had type IVB sequelae of septic arthritis of the hip shows an Ilizarov hip reconstruction osteotomy consisting of proximal valgus osteotomy for pelvic support and distal diaphyseal lengthening for leg length equalization. (*B*) A radiograph taken 2 years after the index operation shows decreased valgus angulation at the proximal osteotomy site. He remains negative for the Trendelenburg sign with an equalized lower limb length after surgery. (*From* Choi IH, Shin YW, Chung CY, et al. Surgical treatment of the severe sequelae of infantile septic arthritis of the hip. Clin Orthop 2005;434:102–9; with permission.)

lescents and young adults. The authors believe, however, that Ilizarov hip reconstruction osteotomy is still indicated if patients are older than 6 years, despite the high probability of repeat pelvic support osteotomy, because second femoral lengthening usually is needed anyway at or near skeletal maturity. The reasons for this belief are that abductor muscle mechanics may further improve with early rather than late Ilizarov hip reconstruction osteotomy and that eliminating a limping gait during the active elementary school period provides a better solution for affected children. If a patient who has type IV sequelae is considered for late Ilizarov hip reconstruction osteotomy for some reason, the importance of hip abductor muscle strengthening exercise together with shoe-lifting for leg-length equalization should be emphasized to the patient on every visit for better outcomes after the Ilizarov surgery.

Adult patients who have a history of infection of the hip in childhood present a challenge as candidates for total hip replacement arthroplasty because of abnormal bone development, soft tissue contractures, the possibility of reinfection, and their relative youth. Kim and colleagues [38] recently reported that there was considerable risk for aseptic loosening because of high prevalence of polyethylene wear and osteolysis that seemed attributable to the less than optimal prosthetic designs and materials used. They reported that there was no recurrence of infection after total hip arthroplasty in patients in whom infection had been quiescent for more than 10 years. One of the concerns regarding Ilizarov hip reconstruction is the potential difficulty of converting to total hip replacement arthroplasty in later life because of the altered anatomy of the proximal femur. These difficulties can be resolved by modern technology, however, because replacement arthroplasty can be used to straighten residual femoral deformity in combination with an osteotomy and the use of a long-stem prosthesis [37].

Summary

When confronted with a child who has severe sequelae, the decision whether to perform a reconstructive or a salvage procedure must be made on an individual basis after considering age, type of sequelae, joint stability and motion, abductor lurch, presence or absence of failed previous reconstructive surgery, and limb-length discrepancy. Ilizarov hip reconstruction should be considered a promising, reliable choice, particularly in older children or young adults who have an unstable but mobile hip caused by the severe sequelae associated with a lower limb-length discrepancy and a Trendelenburg gait.

Ilizarov hip reconstruction not only improves hip biomechanics while preserving hip motion but also equalizes limb-length discrepancies by femoral lengthening. A longer follow-up study in a larger series may provide more complete answers concerning the long-term effectiveness of the technique.

References

[1] Choi IH, Pizzutillo PD, Bowen JR, et al. Sequelae and reconstruction after septic arthritis of the hip in infants. J Bone Joint Surg 1990;72A(8):1150–65.

[2] Betz RR, Cooperman DR, Wopperer JM, et al. Late sequelae of septic arthritis of the hip in infancy and childhood. J Pediatr Orthop 1990;10(3):365–72.

[3] Shaw BA, Kasser JR. Acute septic arthritis in infancy and childhood. Clin Orthop 1990;257:212–25.

[4] Gillespie R. Septic arthritis of childhood. Clin Orthop 1973;96:152–60.

[5] Strong M, Lejman T, Michno P, et al. Sequelae from septic arthritis of the knee during the first 2 years of life. J Pediatr Orthop 1994;14(6):745–51.

[6] Fabry G, Meire E. Septic arthritis of the hip in children: poor results after late and inadequate treatment. J Pediatr Orthop 1983;3(4):461–6.

[7] Hallel T, Salvati EA. Septic arthritis of the hip in infancy: end result study. Clin Orthop 1978;132:115–28.

[8] Hunka L, Said SE, MacKenzie DA, et al. Classification and surgical management of the severe sequelae of septic hips in children. Clin Orthop 1982;171:30–6.

[9] Dobbs MB, Sheridan JJ, Gordon JE, et al. Septic arthritis of the hip in infancy: long-term follow-up. J Pediatr Orthop 2003;23(2):162–8.

[10] Freeland AE, Sullivan DJ, Westin GW. Greater trochanteric hip arthroplasty in children with loss of the femoral head. J Bone Joint Surg 1980;62A(8):1351–61.

[11] Wopperer JM, White JJ, Gillespie R, et al. Long-term follow-up of infantile hip sepsis. J Pediatr Orthop 1988;8(3):322–5.

[12] Choi IH, Shin YW, Chung CY, et al. Surgical treatment of the severe sequelae of infantile septic arthritis of the hip. Clin Orthop 2005;434:102–9.

[13] Wagner H. Osteotomies for congenital hip dislocation. In: The hip, Vol. IV. Proceedings of the fourth open scientific meetings of The Hip Society. St. Louis, MO: CV Mosby; 1976. p. 45–66.

[14] Harmon PH. Surgical treatment of the residual deformity from suppurative arthritis of the hip occurring in young children. J Bone Joint Surg 1942;24(3):576–85.

[15] Colonna PC. A new type of reconstruction operation for old ununited fractures of the neck of the femur. J Bone Joint Surg 1935;17(1):110–22.

[16] Westin GW. The stick femur. In: Proceedings and reports of university colleges, councils and associations. J Bone Joint Surg 1970;52B(4):778–9.

[17] Axer A, Alan A. A new technique for greater trochanteric hip arthroplasty. J Bone Joint Surg 1984;66B(3):331–3.

[18] Weissman SL. Transplantation of the trochanteric epiphysis into the acetabulum after septic arthritis of the hip: report of a case. J Bone Joint Surg 1967;49A(8):1647–51.

[19] Coleman SS. Salvage procedures. In: Congenital dysplasia and dislocation of the hip. St. Louis, MO: CV Mosby; 1978. p. 241–7.

[20] Ilizarov GA. Treatment of disorders of the hip. In: Green SA, editor. Transosseous osteosynthesis. Berlin: Springer Verlag; 1992. p. 668–96.

[21] Catagni MA, Malzev V, Kirienko A. Treatment of disorders of hip joint. In: Maiocchi AB, editor. Advances in Ilizarov apparatus assembly. Milan: Il Quadratino; 1994. p. 119–34.

[22] Paley D. Hip joint considerations. In: Principles of deformity correction. Heidelberg: Springer-Verlag; 2002. p. 647–94.

[23] Kocaoglu M, Eralp L, Sen C, et al. The Ilizarov hip reconstruction osteotomy for hip dislocation. Outcome after 4–7 years in 14 young patients. Acta Orthop Scand 2002;73(4):432–8.

[24] Manzotti A, Rovetta L, Pullen C, et al. Treatment of the late septic arthritis of the hip. Clin Orthop 2003;410:203–12.

[25] Samchukov ML, Birch JG. Pelvic support femoral reconstruction using the method of Ilizarov: a case report. Bull Hosp Joint Dis 1992;52(1):7–11.

[26] Rozbruch SR, Paley D, Bhave A, et al. Ilizarov hip reconstruction for the late sequelae of infantile hip infection. J Bone Joint Surg 2005;87A(5):1007–18.

[27] Lorenz A. Uber die Behandlung der irreponiblen angeborenen Huftluxation und der Schenkelhals peudarthrosen mittels Gabelung (Bifurkation des oberen Femurendes). Wien Klin Wochenschr 1919;32(41):997–9.

[28] Schanz A. Zur Behandlung der veralteten angeborenen Huftverrenkung. Munich Med Wochenschr 1922;69:930–1.

[29] Hass J. Palliative procedures. In: Congenital dislocation of the hip. Springfield, IL: Thomas; 1951. p. 289–307.

[30] Milch H. The pelvic support osteotomy. J Bone Joint Surg 1941;23(3):581–95.

[31] Milch H. The "pelvic support" osteotomy. Clin Orthop 1989;249:4–11.

[32] L'Episcopo J. Stabilization of pathological dislocation of the hip in children. J Bone Joint Surg 1936;18(3):737–42.

[33] Krumins M, Kalnins J, Lacis G. Reconstruction of the proximal end of the femur after hematogenous osteomyelitis. J Pediatr Orthop 1993;13(1):63–7.

[34] Cheng JC, Aguilar J, Leung PC. Hip reconstruction for femoral head loss from septic arthritis in children. A preliminary report. Clin Orthop 1995;314:214–24.

[35] Pauwels F. Biomechanical principles of varus/valgus intertrochanteric osteotomy (Pauwels I and II) in the treatment of osteoarthritis of the hip. In: Schatzker J,

editor. Intertrochanteric osteotomy. Berlin: Springer Verlag; 1983. p. 3–25.

[36] Bombelli R. Structure and function in normal and abnormal hips. 3rd edition. Berlin, Heidelberg: Springer Verlag; 1993. p. 1–55.

[37] Schiltenwolf M, Carstens C, Bernd L, et al. Late results after subtrochanteric angulation osteotomy in young patients. J Pediatr Orthop B 1996;5(4):259–67.

[38] Kim YH, Oh SH, Kim JS. Total hip arthroplasty in adult patients who had childhood infection of the hip. J Bone Joint Surg 2003;85A(2):198–204.

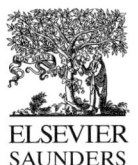

Evaluation and Treatment of Hip Dysplasia in Cerebral Palsy

David A. Spiegel, MD*, John M. Flynn, MD

Division of Orthopaedic Surgery, Children's Hospital of Philadelphia, 2nd Floor Wood Building, 34th Street and Civic Center Boulevard, Philadelphia, PA 19104, USA

Hip problems are commonly identified in patients with cerebral palsy, particularly those with a greater severity of neurologic involvement. Although ambulatory patients with hemiplegia and diplegia typically have torsional abnormalities of the femur, nonambulatory patients with spastic quadriplegia commonly develop neuromuscular hip dysplasia. Pain in the hip region can be a frequent complaint in patients with spastic quadriplegia, and may or may not be secondary to hip subluxation or dislocation.

The focus of this article is the diagnosis and management of neuromuscular hip dysplasia, or "spastic hip disease." Clinical concerns include difficulties with seating or positioning, problems with hygiene and personal care, and occasionally hip pain. The goals of treatment are to maintain a level pelvis; a balanced spine; and mobile, pain-free hips. The natural history is variable, and a large subset of patients develops progressive subluxation of one or both hips, often leading to dislocation. The current approach to treatment focuses on establishing an early diagnosis to prevent these complications. When an early diagnosis is made, nonoperative treatment can be tried to prevent or delay the progression of deformity by maintaining range of motion and decreasing spasticity. In patients with established subluxation or dislocation, goals include improving positioning and ease of care, and treating any discomfort. Surgical options depend on the stage of disease at diagnosis, and may include soft tissue lengthening; reconstructive surgery by soft tissue release combined with a femoral osteotomy with or without a pelvic osteotomy; and salvage procedures, such as resection realignment, or replacement of the femoral head and neck.

Pathophysiology

The progressive changes associated with hip dysplasia in patients with cerebral palsy result from the effects of neuromuscular imbalance on the growth and development of the hip joint [1–4]. The primary problem is spasticity and muscular imbalance, and the musculoskeletal manifestations are secondary.

Soft tissue abnormalities include a muscular imbalance between the stronger flexors and adductors, and the weaker extensors and abductors. With growth, this dynamic imbalance results in myostatic contractures in adduction with or without flexion. These contractures then tether growth, creating progressive changes in the femur and the acetabulum.

Bony abnormalities include femoral torsion with or without coxa valga, and progressive deformity of the femoral head or acetabulum. Most patients have internal femoral torsion (excessive femoral anteversion) caused by inhibition of derotation of the proximal femur during growth. Normal children have approximately 40 degrees of femoral anteversion at birth, which progressively decreases to approximately 15 degrees in the adult. Children with spastic hip disease have a persistence of fetal anteversion, and many have a progressive increase in the degree of anteversion over time. Using a three-dimensional

---

* Corresponding author.
 E-mail address: spiegeld@email.chop.edu (D.A. Spiegel).

finite element model, Shefelbine and Carter [5] predicted a decrease in anteversion angle of 2 degrees per 6 months under normal loading conditions, and an increase of 1 degree per 6 months under the loading conditions typically seen in cerebral palsy. Although many children have a normal femoral neck-shaft angle, a subset has coxa valga. Excessive anteversion may appear to be coxa valga on the anteroposterior radiograph, and a true anteroposterior with anteversion corrected is required to evaluate the neck shaft angle.

A flexion-adduction contracture also shifts the center of rotation of the hip from the femoral head to the lesser trochanter, and the proximal femur is gradually displaced upward and outward [2]. As the femoral head displaces, pressure is concentrated along the posterolateral margin of the acetabulum, which progressively flattens. Asymmetric pressure may deform the femoral head, leading to degeneration of articular cartilage. Pathologic specimens have demonstrated wedging of the epiphysis with focal deformation of the femoral head [6].

In a small subset of patients (1%–2%), usually with extension posturing and hypotonia, the progressive subluxation (or dislocation) is anterior, as is the acetabular deficiency [7,8]. Selva and coworkers [8] found two types of deformity: those with an extension-adduction-external rotation contracture at the hip associated with an extension contracture at the knee, and those with an extension-abduction-external rotation contracture at the hip associated with a flexion deformity at the knee. Fifty percent of patients developed hip pain.

Physical examination

A comprehensive examination includes the spine, hips, and lower extremities. Patients should be evaluated both in their wheelchair and on the examining table. The range of motion at the hips (and lower extremities) is assessed. The spine should be inspected for scoliosis, and if present the location and flexibility are recorded. Sagittal spinal alignment is assessed, and any pelvic obliquity should be noted. On bench examination, a hip flexion deformity can be assessed with the Thomas test. Hip abduction is generally tested with both the hip and the knee in extension. Hip rotation is best assessed with the patient prone. Popliteal angles should also be measured, and the degree of spasticity should be quantified.

With the pelvis viewed as the base of support, the relationship between the hips (infrapelvic alignment) and the spine (suprapelvic alignment) in both the coronal and sagittal plane should be evaluated. In the coronal plane, any pelvic obliquity should be correlated with both the spine and range of motion at the hips. Although the relationship between infrapelvic deformity and scoliosis is debated, several reports have suggested that a primary infrapelvic deformity (adduction contracture) results in pelvic obliquity, and may precede the development of a compensatory lumbar scoliosis with the apex toward the low side of the pelvis [9,10]. On occasion, a lumbar scoliosis with its convexity opposite to the low side of the pelvis may be seen. A primary suprapelvic obliquity (structural scoliosis) also causes pelvic obliquity. In the sagittal plane, although an increase in lumbar lordosis compensates for a hip flexion contracture (causes the pelvis to tilt anteriorly), a lumbar or thoracolumbar kyphosis compensates for an extension contracture of the hip (tight hamstrings, pelvis tilts posteriorly). In these cases, a flexible suprapelvic deformity compensates for the infrapelvic deformity. Although flexion contractures at the hips are less commonly associated with sitting imbalance, significant extension contractures may cause the patient to slide forward in the wheelchair.

In the coronal plane, there may be a windswept appearance of the hips with adduction of one hip and abduction of the other hip, termed the "wind-blown hip" [11]. Electromyographic data suggest that the adductors are active on both sides, whereas the abductors are overactive only on the abducted side [12]. The relationship between suprapelvic and infrapelvic obliquity remains controversial, and the available evidence suggests that infrapelvic obliquity (asymmetric soft tissue contracture) precedes the development of suprapelvic obliquity (scoliosis) [9–11].

Radiologic evaluation

Plain radiographs are commonly used to monitor patients with spastic hip dysplasia. A standardized technique should always be used, with the patient supine and the hip held in neutral adduction-abduction. In patients with a flexion deformity of the hip, the pelvis tilts anteriorly when the hips are extended to obtain the radiograph, which produces an inlet view of the pelvis and makes interpretation difficult. As such, the technician may need maximally to flex the contralateral hip and knee to flatten the lumbar prodosis. The next shaft angle usually appears increased, and "apparent" coxa valga may result from excessive femoral anteversion. Rotation of the hip to correct the excessive anteversion is required to assess accurately the next shaft angle. True coxa valga may also be seen in patients with spastic hip disease.

The migration index is valuable to follow patients for progressive subluxation of the hip. This is calculated by dividing the width of the femoral head that lies outside the lateral margin of the acetabulum (Perkin's line) by the total width of the femoral head (Fig. 1) [13]. In patients without hip disease, the migration percentage is 0% for those less than 4 years of age, and 5% for those 12 to 16 years of age. In the population with cerebral palsy, normal is believed to be less than 30%, whereas subluxation is greater than 30%, and dislocation is greater than 90%. As for other radiographic measurement parameters, there is a normal range of variability. The same technique should be used for all films, and ideally the same observer measures the radiographs, with prior films available for comparison. Reimers [13] believed that a change of 10% represented a true change. More recently, Faraj and coworkers [14] found that for a single observer performing repeated measurements, a 95% confidence interval for a true change was 13%. Parrott and coworkers [15] also reported on the intraobserver (±8% for a true change) and interobserver (±11.6% for a true change) reliability for the migration percentage.

The acetabular index is commonly used to evaluate acetabular dysplasia. The normal acetabular index is 30 degrees at less than 1 year of age, 25 degrees at 1 to 5 years of age, and approximately 20 degrees in an adult. Kay and coworkers [16] found the 95% confidence interval for a true change to be 8 degrees, whereas Spatz and coworkers [17] found an interobserver variability of ±3 degrees and an intraobserver variability of ±3.8 degrees. These exclude variability in pelvic position between radiographs. In spastic hip subluxation, the acetabular index is generally in the range of 40 degrees when the migration index is 50%. Findings on plain radiographs suggest that the acetabular index is normal until approximately 30 months of age, and then becomes progressively higher [18]. It remains unclear whether the acetabulum is shallow [19] or normal [20] in depth. Cooke and coworkers [81] suggested that an acetabular angle of greater than 30 degrees was predictive of dislocation. Although arthrograms are not commonly used in the evaluation of spastic hip disease, Heinrich and coworkers [21] found that the ossification of the lateral pelvic cartilaginous anlage is retarded by progressive subluxation, and was the greatest in hips with a migration index of 52% to 68%.

The morphology of the acetabulum can also be assessed by the shape of the sourcil [22]. The lateral corner is well defined and lies below the weight-bearing dome of the acetabulum in a type I sourcil. In a type II sourcil, the lateral corner is turned upward and lies above the weight-bearing dome. A CT scan of the hips with three-dimensional reconstruction may help to define the nature and location of acetabular deficiency, and on occasion deformity of femoral head also may be identified [19,23,24]. It remains to be determined whether MRI may play a role in evaluating femoral head morphology and cartilage thickness in those subluxated or dislocated hips being considered for reconstructive versus salvage surgery. Although not routine, the authors recommended a CT scan in selected patients in whom acetabular morphology cannot be adequately assessed on plain radiographs.

Natural history

Although the prevalence of hip dysplasia with cerebral palsy varies from 2% to 75%, progressive subluxation is most common in patients with more profound degrees of neurologic involvement [25–28]. Lonstein and Beck [28] identified hip subluxation or dislocation in only 7% of independent ambulators, but in 60% of nonambulators. In the subset of patients who develop progressive dysplasia, the evolution from muscle imbalance to fixed con-

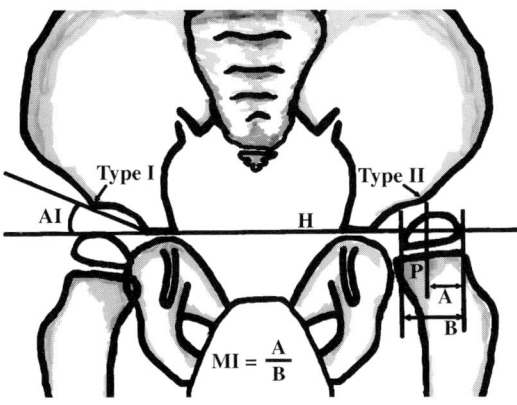

Fig. 1. This illustration demonstrates how to calculate the migration index (MI) and the acetabular index (AI). A type I sourcil lies below the weight-bearing dome of the acetabulum, and the lateral corner is well defined. In a type II sourcil, the lateral corner is turned upward and lies above the weight-bearing dome. H, Hilgenreiner's line; P, Perkin's line. (*From* Flynn JM, Miller F. Management of hip disorders in patients with cerebral palsy. J Am Acad Orthop Surg 2002;10:201; with permission. © 2002 American Academy of Orthopedic Surgeons.)

tracture, subluxation, and finally dislocation usually occurs over several years. Bagg and coworkers [29] found that hips that were stable at 18 years of age remained stable, but that hips with severe subluxation all progressed to dislocation. Miller and Bagg [30] found that although hips with a migration percentage less than 30% were at low risk, those with greater than 60% all became dislocated. The intermediate group had a 25% risk of progression. The results of these studies suggest that close clinical and radiographic follow-up (every 6 months) is required to identify that subset of patients at risk for the development of progressive subluxation or dislocation.

The natural history of the severely subluxated or dislocated hip has also been studied, with variable conclusions. Although several reports have suggested that subluxated or dislocated hips are commonly associated with pain or other problems [27,31,32], which has prompted the current trend toward early screening and aggressive treatment, others have disputed these findings.

Cooperman and coworkers [27] studied 51 dislocated hips with a follow-up of 18 years, and found that half of the dislocated hips were painful. Moreau and coworkers identified hip pain in 11 of 21 institutionalized adults with a dislocated hip [4]. Boldingh and coworkers [31] reviewed 160 patients and found that hip pain was associated with migration and deformity of the femoral head. In contrast, Pritchett [33] studied 80 patients and found that a dislocated hip predisposed to lower-extremity fractures, but did not cause pain, problems with perineal care, or decubitus. The same author reviewed 100 patients with an established dislocation, 50 of whom had surgery for the dislocation, and concluded that there was no difference in outcome, and that pelvic obliquity and scoliosis were related to the degree of neurologic involvement rather than the status of the hips [34]. Knapp and Cortes [35] studied 38 dislocated hips, and found that 18% were definitely painful, whereas 71% were not painful. Noonan and coworkers [36] studied 77 subjects with a mean age of 40 years, of which 15% of the hips were dislocated and 12% were subluxated. Both subluxation and dislocation were associated with radiographic evidence of arthritis, but not necessarily with hip pain. Hip pain and problems with perineal care were identified in patients with less than 30 degrees of hip abduction, with greater than 30 degrees of hip flexion contracture, and with windswept hip deformities.

Chronic musculoskeletal pain is a complaint in up to 67% of adults with cerebral palsy, most commonly in the low back, hip, and leg [37]. Pain in the hip region is commonly encountered in nonambulatory children with spasticity, with or without subluxation or dislocation of one or both hips. The relationship between hip pain and subluxation or dislocation remains elusive in both children and adults. Hodgkinson and coworkers [38] found that the prevalence of pain was 47.2% (tolerable in 35.6%) of 234 nonambulatory adolescents, and that pain could be provoked, linked to position, or spontaneous.

Identifying the source of pain in the region of the hip remains a challenge. Many patients are unable to articulate what they are experiencing, and the clinician must rely on the perception of the parents or caregivers to help identify the source. Pain may be observed at rest, with certain positions, or with such movements as passive abduction. Presumably, pain may originate in the skin or subcutaneous tissues, the musculature surrounding the hip, the osteoarticular structures, or may be referred from another location. Intra-abdominal problems, such as appendicitis, an ovarian cyst, or endometriosis, may present as hip pain. As such, a careful history and physical examination, supplemented by imaging studies or diagnostic injections, may be required to establish the cause and guide treatment. Pain that occurs with passive stretching may be muscular in origin (spasticity with or without contracture), or potentially from hinging of the femoral head on the lateral margin of the acetabulum (or iliac wing) in patients with subluxation or dislocation (with or without breakdown of articular cartilage). Positional pain may result from asymmetric pressure on the skin and subcutaneous tissues, especially in patients with pelvic obliquity caused by suprapelvic (scoliosis) or infrapelvic deformities. Discomfort experienced at rest may be muscular (spasticity), or originate from the articular surface in patients with subluxation or dislocation. On physical examination, the patient's range of motion and response to passive stretching should be assessed.

If a specific pain generator cannot be established despite a careful evaluation, empiric treatment is instituted. Simple measures include avoidance of certain positions, modification of the wheelchair, and nonnarcotic analgesics. When spasticity is believed to play a role, treatment options include oral agents (baclofen, tizanidine); intermuscular injections (botulinum toxin type A, phenol); or intrathecal baclofen. The authors have occasionally performed a diagnostic hip joint injection with a local anesthetic when an intra-articular source is suspected. Further study is required to establish the most appropriate guidelines for the evaluation and treatment of hip pain, and to define better the relationship between radiographic subluxation or dislocation and pain in the pediatric and adolescent population.

Spastic hip disease leading to progressive subluxation with or without dislocation is common in nonambulatory patients with spastic quadriplegia. Although it is clear that a subset of patients with neuromuscular dysplasia have hip pain, the relationship between radiographic findings and clinical findings remains elusive. Patients with progressive dysplasia should be followed closely, and the current trend is to treat these patients early to prevent further subluxation and dislocation. Because hip pain may or may not relate to any observed radiographic changes, a thorough clinical evaluation is suggested to determine the source and to plan treatment.

Nonoperative treatment

An early diagnosis is facilitated by both clinical and radiographic screening, and when there is evidence to suggest that the progression to subluxation and dislocation may be delayed or prevented by early diagnosis and treatment [39,40]. Patients with quadriplegia and marked spasticity should be monitored closely. The authors typically evaluate these patients every 6 months, and focus on the range of motion at the hip. Hips that cannot abduct beyond 30 to 45 degrees (in extension) are believed to be at risk. A baseline radiograph is obtained at 12 to 18 months of age, and the frequency of follow-up radiographs is based on both physical and radiographic findings. When an abduction contracture is present, or the migration percentage is greater than 25%, radiographs may be obtained every 6 months.

The primary problem is in the nervous system, but most treatment strategies have been directed at the end organ. Most of these children receive physical therapy, one goal of which is to maintain the range of motion. Although the effects of physical therapy alone on the natural history of a spastic hip disease remain unknown, efforts to maintain muscle length and prevent contractures should be encouraged. Abduction bracing may be used as an adjunct to stretching, but if used aggressively may cause wind-blown hips or hyperabduction deformity. Achieving compliance with a bracing program may be difficult. Hankinson and Morton [41] performed a prospective trial using a lying hip abduction (20 degrees) system in 14 children with less than 30 degrees abduction before treatment. Six of the 14 abandoned the treatment because of sleep disturbance, and one required surgical intervention. In the seven patients who completed the study, there was an improvement in the migration percentage. Further research is required to determine whether abduction splinting, with or without other therapies, can play a role in altering the natural history of spastic hip disease.

Although passive stretching and splinting are preventive measures directed at the end organ, several recent investigations have addressed the primary problem (spasticity). Intermuscular injection of the adductors with botulinum toxin A has been attempted, and although the psoas is also believed to play an important role in disease progression, the injection is technically more difficulty and has not yet achieved widespread acceptance. The injections need to be repeated at 3- to 6-month intervals, and are accompanied by passive stretching exercises with or without abduction splinting. Pidcock and coworkers [42] looked at the hip migration percentage in 16 patients (9–43 months of age) treated with botulinum toxin A injections to the adductors. Thirteen of these hips started with a migration percentage greater than 30%. At 14 to 49 months follow-up, 18 of 32 patients had a change of 10% or less in the migration percentage, and the greatest improvement was in patients less than 24 months of age with a migration percentage greater than 30%. Boyd and coworkers [43] compared patients treated with botulinum toxin A injections and hip bracing with a group who were observed. At 3 years follow-up, surgery was performed in 47% of patients who did not receive botulinum toxin A, and in 27% of those who did receive botulinum toxin A. Longer-term study is required to determine whether intermuscular injections, with or without other methods of therapy, may alter the natural history. Continuous intrathecal baclofen infusion has been successful in reducing muscle tone in patients with cerebral palsy. In a prospective study by Krach and coworkers [44], 33 patients had an assessment of the migration percentage before and after 1 year of treatment with intrathecal baclofen. A total of 73% of these patients were nonambulatory, and some had had previous orthopedic surgery. The migration percentage remained stable in 91% of patients.

Operative treatment

With the goal of maintaining mobile, located hips to maintain seating balance and prevent pain, surgical treatment is performed in a number of patients with progressive subluxation or dislocation. Operative interventions include soft tissue lengthening [13,45–51]; hip reconstruction by a femoral osteotomy [25,26,52–54] with or without a pelvic osteotomy [3,22,55–63]; or salvage procedures, such as femoral head and neck resection, redirection, or replacement [3,64–74].

Soft tissue procedures have been recommended as a prophylactic measure against bony procedures when the hip is believed to be at risk (passive abduction less than 30–45 degrees, migration percentage greater than 25%), or when there is mild subluxation (migration percentage [MP] > 30%) without coexisting bony deformity. This option may also be considered in children with greater degrees of subluxation who are less than 4 years of age, given the higher risk of recurrence following bony surgery in this population, and as a means to improve motion in patients with greater degrees of deformity who are believed to be at too great a risk for bony surgery.

The goal of soft tissue surgery is to prevent progressive subluxation by rebalancing the muscles (decrease the deforming force in adduction with or without flexion) and restoring motion (relieve myostatic contracture). The specific surgical procedures have varied among published reports, but all authors agree that bilateral procedures should be used to decrease the risk of recurrence or imbalance. Standard components include an open myotomy of the adductor longus and the gracilis, and a partial myotomy of the adductor brevis with greater degrees of contracture. The goal is to achieve at least 30 degrees of passive abduction. Some authors perform routine release or lengthening of the iliopsoas [47,48], whereas others only perform this procedure in the presence of a myostatic contracture [13,45,51]. Obturator neurectomy (anterior branch) remains controversial given the risks of an extension and abduction contracture, and may be indicated in nonambulators with severe spasticity [47,48,75]. An extension and abduction contracture may make it extremely difficult to sit, and may require additional soft tissue releases or shortening femoral osteotomies for adequate seating or positioning [3,8,76,77]. Most authors recommend splinting in abduction (approximately 30 degrees) postoperatively for a variable period of time [37]. Splinting in hyperabduction may predispose to an extension and abduction contracture, especially when an obturator neurectomy has been performed. Several authors have noted better results in patients less than 4 years of age at surgery [13,47], whereas others have suggested that the age at surgery has no bearing on the results [48,51]. Similarly, the migration percentage at the time of surgery may [45,47] or may not [48] predict the outcome.

Presedo and coworkers [48] reviewed the results of a standardized protocol in 129 hips (65 patients, 47 nonambulatory) with 10.8 years follow-up. The indication for an operation was a hip at risk (<45 degrees abduction, MP <25%), and the procedure included myotomy of the adductor longus and gracilis, a release or intramuscular lengthening of the iliopsoas, and an obturator neurectomy in nonambulators. A proximal hamstring release was also performed on occasion. The mean age was 4.4 years, and the postoperative protocol included knee immobilizers and physical therapy. The results were graded as good in 49%, and the failure rate was 30%. Nineteen of 65 children required subsequent bony reconstructive procedures, and a second soft tissue release was required in 11 patients. Overall, the protocol was believed to be effective in 66% of cases. Ambulatory patients had a better outcome than nonambulators, and both the age at surgery and the migration percentage did not affect the outcome. The migration percentage at 1 year postoperatively was predictive of the long-term result. The authors suggest that with early screening and application of a standard protocol, osseous surgery should be required in only 5% of ambulatory and 45% of nonambulatory patients. Cornell and coworkers [45] reviewed 56 hips, and compared patients having a percutaneous release of the adductor longus and gracilis with those treated by an open release including an obturator neurectomy. Success was achieved in 83% when the migration percentage was less than 40%, and there seemed to be no difference between those treated by percutaneous or open techniques. This approach was successful in only 23% of those with a migration percentage of greater than 40%, and failed in all cases with a migration percentage greater than 60%. Reimers [13] found good results following soft tissues releases in 12 of 36 cases. Onimus and coworkers studied 40 hips who were treated at a mean of 4 years of age by myotomy of the adductor longus and gracilis, intramuscular lengthening of the iliopsoas, and obturator neurectomy [47]. At 3-year follow-up, the approach was successful in 67% overall, and in 90% of those less than 4 years of age with a migration percentage less than 33%. Turker and coworkers studied 90 hips treated by myotomy of the adductor longus (±brevis), gracilis, and release of the psoas (50%) with or without obturator neurectomy (or crushing the nerve for temporary denervation) at more than 8 years follow-up [74]. The approach was successful in 42% of patients, and the remaining patients either required additional surgery or developed a dislocation.

In summary, definitive recommendations regarding the efficacy of soft tissue releases are difficult to establish from the existing literature given variations in the patient population (ambulatory and nonambulatory); the indications; the technical details of the procedure; and the postoperative protocols. The results seem to be best when the procedure is performed as a prophylactic measure; however, the lack of a control group in any of these studies makes it difficult to be sure. Stott and Piedrahita [49] published an evidence-based report in which 27 studies involving soft tissue releases for spastic hip disease were scrutinized. Radiographic subluxation was improved in 168 of 530 hips, and the migration percentage was improved in 241 out of 467 hips. Because of the presence of confounding variables (heterogeneity in patient populations, variability in surgical procedures), any conclusions are preliminary and further research is needed to make more specific recommendations.

Osseous reconstruction

Hip reconstruction is considered in patients who have failed soft tissue surgery, or in those who have developed progressive subluxation or dislocation (migration percentage greater than 40%–60%) with or without bony deformity (femoral valgus, acetabular dysplasia). Contraindications to reconstructive surgery include deformity of the femoral head or degenerative changes, and in borderline cases (usually severe subluxation or chronic dislocation) inspection of the femoral head at the time of surgery may be required to decide between reconstruction and salvage. The procedures are tailored to the pathologic findings, and may include a soft tissue release; a proximal femoral varus derotational osteotomy (with or without shortening); a peri-ilial acetabuloplasty; and an open reduction and capsulorrhaphy when necessary (Fig. 2).

For patients presenting without marked deformity of the acetabulum (acetabular index below 25–27 degrees), a proximal femoral varus derotational osteotomy is performed. Components of this procedure include correction of the neck-shaft angle (coxa valga); correction of femoral torsion (persistent fetal anteversion); and shortening of the femur to reduce the muscle forces acting on the hip. A preliminary soft tissue release is performed when passive abduction is less than 45 degrees, because the osteotomy decreases passive abduction. This typically involves the adductor longus, gracilis, and occasionally some fibers of the adductor brevis. If passive abduction remains limited despite these measures, release of the medial capsule may be required. Lengthening or release of the iliopsoas is also performed. In non-ambulators, the psoas tendon may be released when removing a medially based wedge of bone during the osteotomy. In ambulators, the insertion on the lesser trochanter should be preserved, and an intramuscular lengthening may be performed proximally. The appropriate goal for the postoperative neck-shaft angle depends on both age and ambulatory status. If possible, femoral osteotomies should be delayed until at least 4 years of age [52,76]. Mazur and coworkers [76] suggest that remodeling may result in

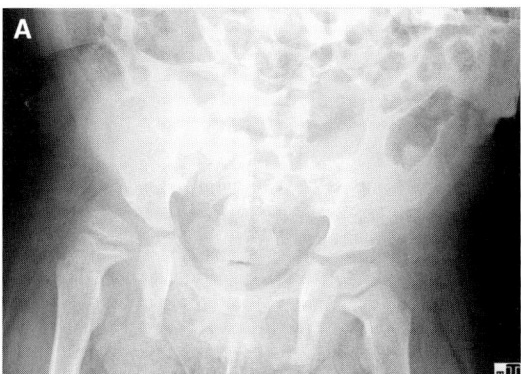 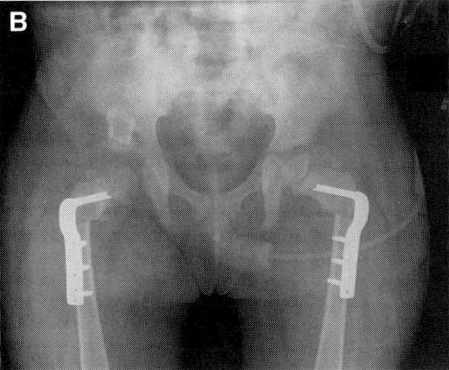

Fig. 2. (A) This 7-year-old boy with spastic quadriplegia had progressive right hip subluxation despite a soft tissue release several years ago. His migration percentage was greater than 70%, and coexisting acetabular dysplasia was present. (B) He underwent bilateral femoral varus derotational osteotomies (family chose bilateral osteotomies to preserve limb length and thigh symmetry), with the goal of a neck-shaft angle of 100 degrees. A volume-reducing pelvic osteotomy was also performed on the right.

a 30-degree increase in neck-shaft angle in children less than 4 years of age, and approximately 20 degrees in patients between 4 and 12 years of age. There was no difference between ambulators and nonambulators. In ambulators, the authors suggest keeping the neck shaft angle between 110 and 120 degrees, depending on the age of the patient, to minimize the chance of abductor insufficiency. In nonambulators, the ideal neck shaft angle varies between 90 and 110 degrees depending on age. Femoral torsion is corrected by externally rotating the distal fragment. Many surgeons choose to fix the osteotomy at a point when there is an even balance between internal and external rotation. Alternatively, a guide pin placed in the femoral neck may be used to estimate both the degree of torsion and the version following derotation. Care should be taken to avoid excessive correction, because retroversion may increase the risk of posterior subluxation or dislocation of the hip. Perhaps the most important component of this procedure is limb shortening, which normalizes the muscle forces acting on the hip. Although the varus osteotomy helps to an extent, it is often beneficial to remove additional bone from the femoral shaft before fixation. The popliteal angle may be used to guide the appropriate amount of bone resected. With the hip flexed to 90 degrees, the amount of overlap at the osteotomy is measured with the popliteal angle at 0 degrees. This amount represents the length of bone that may be removed. The osteotomy is fixed with a small hip screw or a blade plate. Depending on both patient variables (degree of spasticity, bony stock) and the quality of fixation, a spica cast may be desirable for at least several weeks postoperatively. Some surgeons prefer to perform bilateral femoral osteotomies with the goal of equalizing limb lengths and muscle balance about the hips. If unilateral surgery is performed, there is an asymmetry in the appearance of the proximal thigh and in leg lengths. Whether the prevalence of recurrent deformity is greater following unilateral bony surgery remains to be determined.

Patients with coexisting acetabular dysplasia (acetabular index >25 degrees, type II sourcil) require a pelvic osteotomy. In most spastic subluxation cases, the acetabular deficiency is posterolateral or global. Because the acetabulum is typically shallow and saucer shaped, the most common procedures in patients with neuromuscular hip dysplasia are volume-reducing procedures rather than redirectional procedures. Although some authors have reported success with a Pemberton osteotomy [55,62], most have performed variants of the osteotomy described by Dega [3,22,56–58,60,61,63]. A pericapsular osteotomy is performed approximately 5 mm above the insertion of the joint capsule. The cuts are visualized using an image intensifier, and curved osteotomies are required. The osteotomy extends down to the triradiate cartilage, which serves as a hinge. The lateral margin of the acetabulum is then levered downward, and triangular bone grafts are inserted. Several options are available for graft material, including tricortical iliac crest allograft, triangular grafts from the iliac crest, or a triangular wedge of bone removed during the femoral osteotomy. The location of insertion may be used to maximize coverage in one area. Variations in technique typically surround whether or not the osteotomy is extended into the sciatic notch, and whether a bicortical cut is made anteriorly. Fixation is not required, and a spica cast is not mandatory. For patients with greater degrees of subluxation or dislocation, an open reduction also may be required. The indications for open reduction are variable, and the San Diego group has suggested that a migration percentage of greater than 70% is an indication for routine open reduction [57,58]. Miller and coworkers [22] have suggested doing a medial capsulotomy if there is less than 20 degrees of abduction and the femoral head does not reduce under the acetabulum after the pelvic osteotomy.

Postoperatively, both diazepam and narcotics are generally required. Complications include a variety of medical problems (pneumonia, atelectasis, urinary tract infection); pressure sores; heterotopic ossification (increased risk if spine fusion is performed within 6 weeks) [78]; avascular necrosis of the femoral head; and insufficiency fractures. Stasikelis and coworkers [79] found that complications developed in 68% of patients with spastic quadriplegia and a gastrostomy or tracheostomy tube (12% without) and in 29% of nonambulators (8% of ambulators).

McNerney and coworkers [57] reported the results of a combined reconstruction of 104 hips with a mean follow-up of 6.9 years. The indications for a pelvic osteotomy included an open triradiate cartilage, an acetabular index greater than 25 degrees, and a migration percentage greater than 40%. An open reduction was routinely performed when the migration percentage exceeded 70%. Ninety-five percent of the hips remained well reduced at follow-up and there were no redislocations. Eight percent developed avascular necrosis. Miller and coworkers [22] reviewed 49 subluxated and 21 dislocated hips treated by a single-stage reconstruction including soft tissue releases, a femoral osteotomy, and in most cases a volume-reducing pelvic osteotomy. At 34 months follow-up, all but two hips remained located, 82% of patients with hip pain had complete relief, there were no cases of avascular necrosis and 80% of caretakers believed that the surgery had been of benefit.

For symptomatic, older patients with subluxation or dislocation in whom deformity of the femoral head or degenerative changes preclude hip reconstruction, several options are available for salvage. The decision between reconstruction and salvage is often made intraoperatively by direct inspection of the femoral head. There is no consensus regarding the optimal treatment for this difficult problem, and options include resection of the femoral head and neck; valgus osteotomy; femoral shortening osteotomy; resection, valgus, soft tissue interposition (McHale procedure); arthrodesis; and arthroplasty (total hip versus humeral prosthesis).

The technique of proximal femoral resection-interposition arthroplasty was initially described by Castle and Schneider [66], and involves an extraperiosteal resection of the proximal femur just below the lesser trochanter. The quadriceps muscle is sutured down over the femoral shaft, and both the joint capsule and the abductors are sutured down over the acetabulum. Postoperative Russell traction was used until soft tissue healing was complete. Several studies have reported adequate results following this procedure [64,66,70,74]. Postoperative concerns include the formation of heterotopic ossification and proximal migration of the femoral shaft. McCarthy and coworkers [70] modified this slightly by using a line across the distal ischia to define the level of resection, and used 90-90 skeletal traction for 6 weeks. They reviewed 56 hips in 34 patients after a minimum of 2 years and found that all patients had an improvement in motion, and all but one had an improvement in seating. Heterotopic bone was identified in most patients; however, additional surgery was only required in a small subset. Widmann and coworkers [74] reviewed 18 hips treated in this fashion, most of which had prior surgical procedures. At more than 7 years follow-up, all patients exhibited adequate pain relief, improvement in motion, and improvement in seating. Postoperative irradiation was successful in decreasing heterotopic ossification, and skin traction was as effective as skeletal traction in preventing proximal migration. Pain relief was maximal at an average of more than 5 months following the procedure. These results suggest that proximal femoral resection-interposition arthroplasty remains a good option for salvage. Care should be taken to minimize soft tissue trauma during the dissection, to maintain adequate hemostasis, and to use suction drainage postoperatively. Postoperative irradiation should be considered, and skin traction may be as effective as skeletal traction.

The McHale procedure involves an adductor release; a resection of the femoral head and neck at the level of the base of the femoral neck; a valgus proximal femoral osteotomy with plate fixation (to achieve 45-degree abduction); placement of the lesser trochanter into the acetabulum (suture the psoas tendon to the ligamentum teres); and a capsulorrhaphy [71]. Patients were placed in a spica cast for approximately 3 weeks. There was improvement in pain, range of motion, and sitting endurance in all five patients. One patient exhibited a small amount of heterotopic ossification, and there was no proximal migration. In a retrospective review of 36 hips, Leet and coworkers [69] compared the McHale procedure with proximal femoral head resection (postoperative traction or an external fixator to maintain length). The age at surgery was 19 years, and the average follow up was 3.4 years. Although both groups had an improvement in their pain and an increase in their sitting tolerance, those treated by the McHale procedure had a shorter length of stay, lower rate of complications, and decreased superior migration of the femoral head.

Other alternatives described in a limited number of studies include femoral shortening osteotomy [80], hip arthrodesis [67], and prosthetic reconstruction [65,68,72,73]. Terjesen and Hellum [80] performed a femoral shortening osteotomy (3–5 cm) at the subtrochanteric level in 15 patients with chronic dislocations, and found adequate symptomatic relief in all patients at 5 years follow-up. Five of the 16 hips were reduced at follow-up. Arthrodesis of the hip has been reported in a limited number of patients, and may be considered in nonambulatory patients with unilateral disease [68]. Prosthetic reconstruction has also been reported, most commonly in ambulatory patients with painful degenerative changes [65,72,73]. Buly and coworkers [65] reviewed 18 adults treated by a cemented total hip arthroplasty at 10 years follow-up. A spica cast was used in the immediate postoperative period. Pain relief was achieved in 94%, and at latest follow-up 95% had no evidence of loosening. Weber and Cabanela [73] reviewed 16 patients following total hip arthroplasty, and found adequate pain relief in 87%, with an improvement in function in 79%. Gabos and coworkers [68] implanted a noncemented humeral prosthesis in 14 hips (11 patients) with degenerative arthritis. In seven hips a glenoid component was inserted into the false acetabulum. At 5 years follow-up, 10 of 11 patients had complete pain relief, although four prostheses became dislocated. Caregiver satisfaction with seating and motion was high. Five patients developed heterotopic ossification, and one implant exhibited osteolysis.

Summary

Hip problems are very common in patients with cerebral palsy, particularly those who are nonambulatory with a large degree of spasticity. The emphasis has been on early detection of patients at risk for progressive dysplasia, and both clinical and radiographic screening may be useful for early detection. Although the natural history is variable, and not all hips progress to subluxation or dislocation, a subset of patients with chronically subluxated or dislocated hips has discomfort. Nonoperative strategies are currently under investigation, and it remains unclear whether physical therapy, abduction splinting, botulinum toxin A, or interthecal baclofen alter the natural history of spastic hip disease. For patients with early disease and the absence of bony deformity, a soft tissue release may play a role in stabilizing the hip. For those with established deformity, reconstructive or salvage options are available depending on the shape of the femoral head and the status of the articular cartilage. Reconstructive surgery usually involves a soft tissue release followed by a proximal femoral varus derotational osteotomy. Patients with coexisting acetabular dysplasia benefit from a volume-reducing pelvic osteotomy. A subset of patients may also benefit from an open reduction and capsulotomy, and this also facilitates inspection of the femoral head. For patients with established dislocation, or severe subluxation with deformity of the femoral head and breakdown of articular cartilage, a host of salvage options are available.

References

[1] Bleck EE. The hip in cerebral palsy. Orthop Clin North Am 1980;11:79–104.

[2] Drummond DS, Rogala EJ, Cruess R, et al. The paralytic hip in pelvic obliquity in cerebral palsy and myelodysplasia. AAOS Instr Course Lect 1979;28:7–36.

[3] Flynn JM, Miller F. Management of hip disorders in patients with cerebral palsy. J Am Acad Orthop Surg 2002;10:198–209.

[4] Moreau M, Drummond DS, Rogala E, et al. Natural history of the dislocated hip in spastic cerebral palsy. Dev Med Child Neurol 1979;21:749–53.

[5] Shefelbine SJ, Carter DR. Mechanobiological predictions of femoral anteversion in cerebral palsy. Ann Biomed Eng 2004;32:297–305.

[6] Lundy DW, Ganey TM, Ogden JA, et al. Pathologic morphology of the dislocated proximal femur in children with cerebral palsy. J Pediatr Orthop 1998;18:528–34.

[7] Bowen JR, MacEwen GD, Mathews PA. Treatment of extension contracture of the hip in cerebral palsy. Dev Med Child Neurol 1981;23:23–9.

[8] Selva G, Miller F, Dabney KW. Anterior hip dislocation in children with cerebral palsy. J Pediatr Orthop 1998;18:54–61.

[9] Abel MF, Blanco JS, Pavlovich L, et al. Asymmetric hip deformity and subluxation in cerebral palsy: an analysis of surgical treatment. J Pediatr Orthop 1999;19:479–85.

[10] Black BE, Griffin PP. The cerebral palsied hip. Clin Orthop 1997;338:42–51.

[11] Letts M, Shapiro L, Mulder K, et al. The windblown hip syndrome in total body cerebral palsy. J Pediatr Orthop 1984;4:55–62.

[12] Nwaobi OM, Sussman MD. Electromyographic and force patterns of cerebral palsy patients with windblown hip deformity. J Pediatr Orthop 1990;10:382–8.

[13] Reimers J. The stability of the hip in children: a radiological study of the results of muscle surgery in cerebral palsy. Acta Orthop Scand Suppl 1980;184:1–100.

[14] Faraj S, Atherton WG, Stott NS. Inter-and intra-measurer error in the measurement of Reimer's hip migration percentage. J Bone Joint Surg Br 2004;86:434–7.

[15] Parrott J, Boyd RN, Dobson F, et al. Hip displacement in spastic cerebral palsy: repeatability of radiologic measurement. J Pediatr Orthop 2002;22:660–7.

[16] Kay RM, Watts HG, Dorey FJ. Variability in the assessment of the acetabular index. J Pediatr Orthop 1997;17:170–3.

[17] Spatz DK, Reiger M, Klaumann M, et al. Measurement of acetabular index intraobserver and interobserver variation. J Pediatr Orthop 1997;17:174–5.

[18] Cornell MS. The hip in cerebral palsy. Dev Med Child Neurol 1995;37:3–18.

[19] Abel MF, Wenger DR, Mubarak SJ, et al. Quantitative analysis of hip dysplasia in cerebral palsy: a study of radiographs and 3-D reformatted images. J Pediatr Orthop 1994;14:283–9.

[20] Brunner R, Picard C, Robb J. Morphology of the acetabulum in hip dislocations caused by cerebral palsy. J Pediatr Orthop B 1997;6:207–11.

[21] Heinrich SD, MacEwen GD, Zembo MM. Hip dysplasia, subluxation, and dislocation in cerebral palsy: an arthrographic analysis. J Pediatr Orthop 1991;11:488–93.

[22] Miller F, Girardi H, Lipton G, et al. Reconstruction of the dysplastic spastic hip with peri-ilial pelvic and femoral osteotomy followed by immediate mobilization. J Pediatr Orthop 1997;17:592–602.

[23] Buckley SL, Sponseller PD, Magid D. The acetabulum in congenital and neuromuscular hip instability. J Pediatr Orthop 1991;11:498–501.

[24] Kim HT, Wenger DR. Location of acetabular deficiency and associated hip dislocation in neuromuscular hip dysplasia: three-dimensional computed tomographic analysis. J Pediatr Orthop 1997;17:143–51.

[25] Brunner R, Baumann JU. Clinical benefit of reconstruction of dislocated or subluxated hip joints in patients with spastic cerebral palsy. J Pediatr Orthop 1994;14:290–4.

[26] Carr C, Gage JR. The fate of the nonoperated hip in cerebral palsy. J Pediatr Orthop 1987;7:262–7.

[27] Cooperman DR, Bartucci E, Dietrick E, et al. Hip dislocation in spastic cerebral palsy: long term consequences. J Pediatr Orthop 1987;7:268–76.

[28] Lonstein JE, Beck K. Hip dislocation and subluxation in cerebral palsy. J Pediatr Orthop 1986;6:521–6.

[29] Bagg MR, Farber J, Miller F. Long-term follow-up of hip subluxation in cerebral palsy patients. J Pediatr Orthop 1993;13:32–6.

[30] Miller F, Bagg MR. Age and migration percentage as risk factors for progression in spastic hip disease. Dev Med Child Neurol 1995;37:449–55.

[31] Boldingh EJ, Jacobs-van der Bruggen MA, Bos CF, et al. Determinants of hip pain in adult patients with severe cerebral palsy. J Pediatr Orthop 2005;14:120–5.

[32] Houkom JA, Roach JW, Wenger DR, et al. Treatment of acquired hip subluxation in cerebral palsy. J Pediatr Orthop 1986;6:285–90.

[33] Pritchett JW. The untreated unstable hip in severe cerebral palsy. Clin Orthop Rel Res 1983;173:169–72.

[34] Pritchett JW. Treated and untreated unstable hips in cerebral palsy. Dev Med Child Neurol 1990;32:3–6.

[35] Knapp DR, Cortes H. Untreated hip dislocation in cerebral palsy. J Pediatr Orthop 2002;22:668–71.

[36] Noonan KJ, Walker TL, Kayes KJ, et al. Effect of surgery on the nontreated hip in severe cerebral palsy. J Pediatr Orthop 2000;20:771–5.

[37] Engel JM, Jensen MP, Hoffman AJ, et al. Pain in persons with cerebral palsy: extension and cross validation. Arch Phys Med Rehabil 2003;84:1125–8.

[38] Hodgkinson I, Jindrich ML, Duhaut P, et al. Hip pain in 234 nonambulatory adolescents and young adults with cerebral palsy: a cross sectional multi center study. Dev Med Child Neurol 2001;43:806–8.

[39] Dobson F, Boyd RN, Parrott J, et al. Hip surveillance in children with cerebral palsy: impact on the surgical management of spastic hip disease. J Bone Joint Surg Br 2005;84:720–6.

[40] Hagglund G, Andersson S, Lauge-Peterson H, et al. Prevention of dislocation of the hip in children with cerebral palsy: the first ten years of a population-based prevention program. J Bone Joint Surg Br 2005;87:95–101.

[41] Hankinson J, Morton RE. Use of a lying hip abduction system in children with bilateral cerebral palsy: a pilot study. Dev Med Neurol 2002;44:177–80.

[42] Pidcock FS, Fish DE, Johnson-Greene D, et al. Hip migration percentage in children with cerebral palsy treated with Botulinum toxin A. Arch Phys Med Rehabil 2005;86:431–5.

[43] Boyd RN, Dobson F, Parrott J, et al. The effect of botulinum toxin A and a variable hip abduction orthosis on gross motor function: a randomized controlled trial. Eur J Neurol 2001;8(Suppl 5):109–19.

[44] Krach LE, Kriel RL, Gilmartin RC, et al. Hip status in cerebral palsy after one year of continuous intrathecal baclofen infusion. Pediatr Neurol 2004;30:163–8.

[45] Cornell MS, Hatrick NC, Boyd R, et al. The hip in children with cerebral palsy: predicting the outcome of soft tissue surgery. Clin Orthop 1997;340:165–71.

[46] Miller F, Slomczykowski M, Cope R, et al. Computer modeling of the pathomechanics of spastic hip dislocation in children. J Pediatr Orthop 1999;19:486–92.

[47] Onimus M, Allamel G, Manzone P, et al. Prevention of hip dislocation in cerebral palsy by early psoas and adductor tenotomies. J Pediatr Orthop 1991;11:432–5.

[48] Presedo A, Chang-Wug O, Dabney KW, et al. Soft-tissue releases to treat spastic hip subluxation in children with cerebral palsy. J Bone Joint Surg Am 2005;87:832–41.

[49] Stott NS, Piedrahita L. Effects of surgical adductor releases for hip subluxation in cerebral palsy: an AACPDM evidence report. Dev Med Child Neurol 2004;46:628–45.

[50] Terjesen T, Lie GD, Hyldmo AA, et al. Adductor tenotomy in spastic cerebral palsy: a long term follow-up study of 78 patients. Acta Orthop 2005;76:128–37.

[51] Turker RJ, Lee R. Adductor tenotomies in children with quadriplegic cerebral palsy: longer term followup. J Pediatr Orthop 2000;20:370–4.

[52] Brunner R, Baumann JU. Long-term effects of intertrochanteric varus derotation osteotomy on femur and acetabulum in spastic cerebral palsy: an 11- to 18-year follow-up study. J Pediatr Orthop 1997;17:585–91.

[53] Hoffer MM. Management of the hip in cerebral palsy. J Bone Joint Surg Am 1986;68:629–31.

[54] Noonan KJ, Walker TL, Kayes KJ, et al. Varus derotational osteotomy for the treatment of hip subluxation and dislocation in cerebral palsy: statistical analysis in 73 hips. J Pediatr Orthop B 2001;10:279–86.

[55] Gordon JE, Capelli AM, Strecker WB, et al. Pemberton pelvic osteotomy and varus rotational osteotomy in the treatment of acetabular dysplasia in patients who have static encephalopathy. J Bone Joint Surg Am 1996;78:1863–71.

[56] Jozwiak M, Marciniak W, Piontek T, et al. Dega's transiliac osteotomy in the treatment of spastic hip subluxation and dislocation in cerebral palsy. J Pediatr Orthop B 2000;9:257–64.

[57] McNerney NP, Mubarak SJ, Wenger DR. One-stage correction of the dysplastic hip in cerebral palsy with the San Diego acetabuloplasty: results and complications in 104 hips. J Pediatr Orthop 2000;20:93–103.

[58] Mubarak SJ, Valencia FG, Wenger DR. One-stage correction of the spastic dislocated hip: use of pericapsular acetabuloplasty to improve coverage. J Bone Joint Surg Am 1992;74:1347–57.

[59] Owers KL, Pyman J, Gargan MF, et al. Bilateral hip surgery in cerebral palsy: a preliminary review. J Bone Joint Surg Br 2001;83:1161–7.

[60] Root L, Laplaza FJ, Brourman SN, et al. The severely unstable hip in cerebral palsy: treatment with open reduction, pelvic osteotomy, and femoral osteotomy with shortening. J Bone Joint Surg Am 1995;77:703–12.

[61] Roposch A, Wedge JH. An incomplete periacetabular osteotomy for treatment of neuromuscular hip dysplasia. Clin Orthop Rel Res 2005;431:166–75.

[62] Shea KG, Coleman SS, Carroll K, et al. Pemberton pericapsular osteotomy to treat a dysplastic hip in cerebral palsy. J Bone Joint Surg Am 1997;79:1342–51.

[63] Song HR, Carroll NC. Femoral varus derotation osteotomy with or without acetabuloplasty for unstable hips in cerebral palsy. J Pediatr Orthop 1998;18:62–8.

[64] Baxter MP, D'Astous JL. Proximal femoral resection-interposition arthroplasty: salvage hip surgery for the severely disabled child with cerebral palsy. J Pediatr Orthop 1986;6:681–6.

[65] Buly RL, Huo M, Root L, et al. Total hip arthroplasty in cerebral palsy: long-term follow-up results. Clin Orthop 1993;296:148–53.

[66] Castle ME, Schneider C. Proximal femoral resection-interposition arthroplasty. Bone Joint Surg Am 1978;60:1051–4.

[67] deMoraes Barros Fucs PM, Svartman C, de Assumpcao RMC, et al. Treatment of the painful chronically dislocated and subluxated hip in cerebral palsy with hip arthrodesis. J Pediatr Orthop 2003;23:529–34.

[68] Gabos PG, Miller F, Galban MA, et al. Prosthetic interposition arthroplasty for the palliative treatment of end-stage spastic hip disease in nonambulatory patients with cerebral palsy. J Pediatr Orthop 1999;19:796–804.

[69] Leet AI, Chhor K, Launay F, et al. Femoral head resection for painful hip subluxation in cerebral palsy: Is valgus osteotomy in conjunction with femoral head resection preferable to proximal femoral head resection and traction? J Pediatr Orthop 2005;25:70–3.

[70] McCarthy RE, Simon S, Douglas B, et al. Proximal femoral resection to allow adults who have severe cerebral palsy to sit. J Bone Joint Surg Am 1988;70:1011–6.

[71] McHale KA, Bagg M, Nason SS. Treatment of the chronically dislocated hip in adolescents with cerebral palsy with femoral head resection and subtrochanteric valgus osteotomy. J Pediatr Orthop 1990;10:504–9.

[72] Root L, Goss JR, Mendes J. The treatment of the painful hip in cerebral palsy by total hip replacement or hip arthrodesis. J Bone Joint Surg Am 1986;68:590–8.

[73] Weber M, Cabanela ME. Total hip arthroplasty in patients with cerebral palsy. Orthopaedics 1999;22:425–7.

[74] Widmann RF, Do TT, Doyle SM, et al. Resection arthroplasty of the hip for patients with cerebral palsy: an outcome study. J Pediatr Orthop 1999;19:805–10.

[75] Matsuo T, Tada S, Hajime T. Insufficiency of the hip adductor after anterior obturator neurectomy in 42 children with cerebral palsy. J Pediatr Orthop 1986;6:686–92.

[76] Mazur JM, Danko AM, Standard SC, et al. Remodelling of the proximal femur after varus osteotomy in children with cerebral palsy. Dev Med Child Neurol 2004;46:412–5.

[77] Szalay EA, Roach JW, Houkom JA, et al. Extension-abduction contracture of the spastic hip. J Pediatr Orthop 1986;6:1–6.

[78] Krum SD, Miller F. Heterotopic ossification after hip and spine surgery in children with cerebral palsy. J Pediatr Orthop 1993;13:739–43.

[79] Stasikelis PJ, Lee DD, Sullivan CM. Complications of osteotomies in severe cerebral palsy. J Pediatr Orthop 1999;19:207–10.

[80] Terjesen T, Hellum C. Femoral shortening osteotomy for chronic hip dislocation in patients with cerebral palsy. Tidsskr Nor Laegeforen 1998;118:2773–6.

[81] Cooke PH, Cole WG, Carey RP. Dislocation of the hip in cerebral palsy: natural history and predictability. J Bone Joint Surg Br 1989;71:441–6.

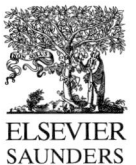

Hip Disorders in Children Who Have Spinal Cord Injury

James J. McCarthy, MD[a,b,*], Randal R. Betz, MD[a,b]

[a]*Shriners Hospital for Children–Philadelphia, 3551 North Broad Street, Philadelphia, PA 19140, USA*
[b]*Department of Orthopaedic Surgery, Temple University, 3551 North Broad Street, Philadelphia, PA 19140, USA*

Little has been written regarding the assessment and treatment of hip disorders in children who have underlying paralysis. This may be because of the small number of children who have spinal cord injuries. Each year approximately 2000 people younger than 20 years of age suffer a spinal cord injury (SCI) [1]; most of these are older at the time of injury. This compares with a larger number of children who have other forms of neurologic disorders, such as myelodysplasia, which affects approximately 6000 newborns annually in the United States, and for which there is a large body of literature describing the natural history and treatment of hip disorders in children who have myelodysplasia [2]. This article focuses only on hip disorders in children who have SCI, although there is clearly commonality in hip disorders that transcends many neurologic disorders.

The underlying treatment principle for all children who have SCI is prevention. This includes appropriate car seats and restraints and avoidance of activities or techniques that could result in an SCI. Treatment of the acute child who has SCI is evolving, and new research aimed at spinal cord regeneration is ongoing. Despite this, the current treatment focus of the orthopedic surgeon is on rehabilitation and prevention of deformity. Decision treatments can be difficult because of the limited amount of information regarding this patient population and the long-term natural history, the diversity of the clinical presentation, and the hope of significant future treatment breakthroughs.

Disorders that affect children who have SCI include hip subluxation and dislocation, hip contractures, heterotopic ossification, sepsis, and fractures. Other disorders less commonly described include joint space narrowing and bony destruction of unknown etiology. This article describes the evaluation and treatment of children who have paralytic hip disorders.

Hip subluxation/dislocation

Hip subluxation and dislocation is common in the child who has SCI. Hip subluxation is a radiographic diagnosis that refers to the loss of full containment of the femoral head within the bony acetabulum and usually is measured by a percentage or degree of subluxation, referred to as the migration index (Fig. 1) [3]. As this number or percent increases, there is a gradual loss of bony contact until at 100% uncovering there is no contact between the femoral head and acetabulum, and the term dislocated is used. In children who have a spinal cord injury this typically occurs gradually over several years, but there are exceptions. Although uncommon, hip dislocations can occur from trauma at the time of injury. The diagnosis and treatment of this is similar to any acute, traumatic hip dislocation. The etiology of hip subluxation or dislocation in SCI can be underlying sepsis. Unlike children or adults who are sensate, the clinical findings can be subtle and may include systemic manifestations, such as a generalized increase in spasticity or symptoms of autonomic dysreflexia. The prompt diagnosis and treatment of this condition is critical, because an untreated septic hip can result

No financial support was received for this manuscript.
* Corresponding author. Shriners Hospital for Children–Philadelphia, 3551 North Broad Street, Philadelphia, PA 19140.
E-mail address: JMcCarthy@shrinenet.org (J.J. McCarthy).

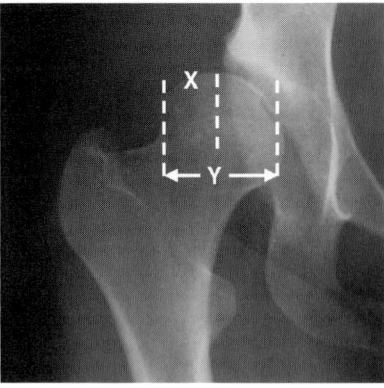

Fig. 1. The migration index. (*From* Reimers J. The stability of the hip in children. A radiological study of the results of muscle surgery in cerebral palsy. Acta Orthop Scand 1980;184(Suppl):1–100; with permission.)

in total destruction of the joint. Radiographically, there may be few signs. Frank hip dislocation is a late finding, although an increase in the medial joint space or changes in the density of the soft tissues may be noticed. If there is any concern, laboratory evaluation for signs of infection should be sought and hip joint aspiration performed.

Nonseptic hip subluxation or dislocation can be associated with a spastic paralysis or flaccid paralysis and rarely is noticed clinically unless the hip is completely dislocated [4]. The reported incidence of nonseptic hip subluxation or dislocation in children who have SCI varies from 29% to 82% and seems related to age at the time of injury [5–7] and to other factors, such as degree of tone [8]. Rink reported on 17 patients, all 9 years of age or younger at the time of SCI, and found that 14 patients (82%) had developed subluxation or dislocation of one or more of their hips [6]. Vogel and colleagues [7,9] have shown an association between age of injury and hip subluxation. In a presentation to the annual American Spinal Injury Association Meeting [10], they found that 66% of patients between birth and 4 years of age at the time of injury had an unstable hip. The incidence decreased with increasing age at the time of injury so that only 6% of those who were between 13 and 21 years of age at the time of injury had an unstable hip. Pierre-Jacques and colleagues [11] reported an overall rate of hip instability of 43% (31 of 72 hips). Of those 31, 22 were subluxed and 9 were dislocated, and most of the patients had spastic paralysis (25 of 31 hips, or 80%) versus flaccid paralysis (6 of 31, or 21%). The authors' study found that 48% of children who had SCI had at least one hip with subluxation/dislocation, but that 93% of children who had onset of injury at or before age 10 years had hip subluxation/dislocation, whereas only 9% of children who were older than age 10 years at the time of injury did. Other radiographic findings were noticed in approximately one third of the patients on follow-up radiographs, however, including complete radiographic destruction (of unknown etiology), decreased superior joint space (≤ 2 mm), fractures of the hip or femur, and heterotopic ossification. Most of these occurred in children who were older than age 10 years at the time injury [5] (Fig. 2).

For the patient who has an SCI that occurs at a young age, especially patients 10 years and younger, an aggressive prevention approach is strongly recommended. This includes active soft tissue stretching, control of spasticity, and prophylactic abduction bracing. In this group, the authors recommend bracing at night, keeping the hips in an abducted position, and if they use a wheelchair, fitting it with a pummel to keep the hips abducted while sitting.

Surgical treatment for hip subluxation and dislocation is more controversial. The indications for surgical treatment of hip instability, once established, are less clear. Traditionally most centers and most investigators recommend no treatment for hip subluxation or dislocation in children, as it is believed to have little functional implication with regard to ambulation for patients who require bracing. Rink and

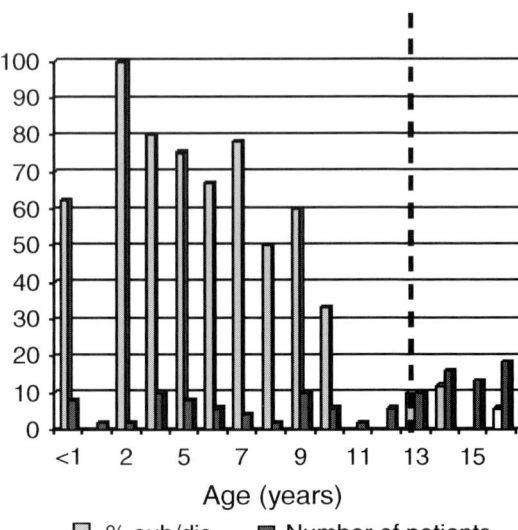

Fig. 2. Percentage of hips subluxed or dislocated plotted against age; 93% of those ≤ 10 years old at the time of the SCI had dislocated hips, versus only 9% of those >10 years old.

colleagues [6] evaluated 17 children younger than age 9 years at the time of SCI with hip subluxation or dislocation and found no ambulatory changes, although one patient developed pain and three had evidence of avascular necrosis. The authors also reported little functional benefit to hip reduction after surgery in children who have SCI [4]. Unfortunately the implications of hip subluxation or dislocation as an adult seem less benign. Two investigators have reported on the association of hip dislocation and autonomic dysreflexia in adult patients with SCI [12]. Baird and colleagues [13] reported on 11 adults who had SCI and found that 5 had pain, 5 had decreased sitting tolerance, and 3 had an increase in skin ulcerations.

Also confusing the surgical indications is the growing number of established research programs in spinal cord regeneration showing promising results and, similarly, research programs with functional electrical stimulation (FES) for standing and upright mobility [14]. For patients for whom spinal cord regeneration or FES may be options, treatment of hip instability may be advisable. In one study, Betz and colleagues [15] found that a located hip is critical for functional electrical stimulation (FES) assisted mobility.

Further adding to the confusion is the dearth of information regarding the results of surgical treatment for children who have SCI. The authors reported on the results of 21 hips in 13 patients at an average 33-month follow-up [4] and found that the degree of subluxation (migration index) improved from a mean of 44% preoperatively to 1% after surgery, although it increased slowly to a mean of 19% at follow-up. Functional scores (by way of the functional independence measure, or FIM) improved but did not reach statistic significance, and no patient lost range of motion such that it interfered with activities. Complications included skin problems and fractures (two patients). It is important to emphasize that treatment of longstanding dislocations, especially if there are bony articular changes, is not advisable. As we gain more insight into the techniques and results of surgical reduction and with regeneration strategies and FES becoming available in the future, more aggressive hip stability management may be recommended.

If surgical treatment of hip subluxation or dislocation is chosen, as a general guideline patients who have spastic hip instability can be treated similarly to those patients who have cerebral palsy, and patients who have flaccid paralysis can be treated similarly to those who have spina bifida. Other guiding principles include correction of soft-tissue contractures, muscle balancing, and correction of bony instability.

Treatment of hip dislocation or subluxation in children who have spastic SCI generally requires controlling the spasticity first. Surgical correction involves performing needed soft-tissue releases of any contractures and then bony procedures. The type of bony procedure is determined based on the ana-

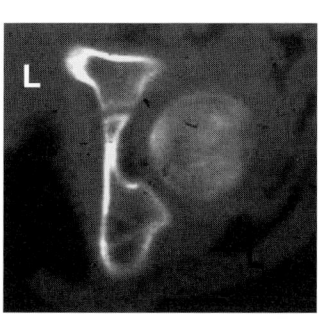
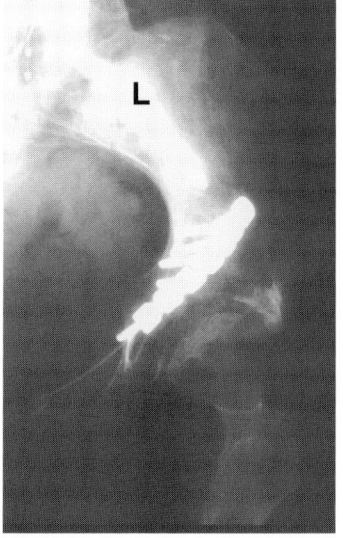
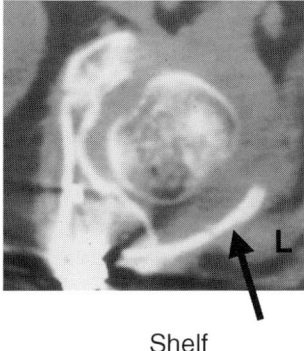

Fig. 3. The posterior shelf operation.

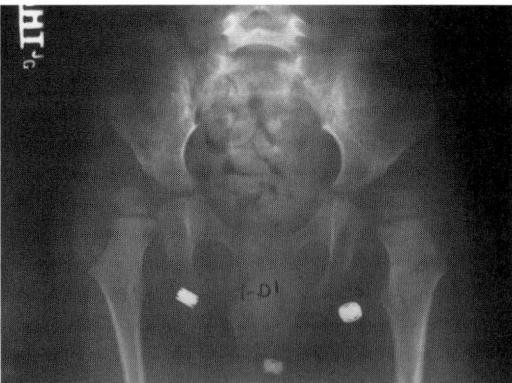

Fig. 4. An AP radiograph of the pelvis of a 4-year-old child who had a T4 incomplete spinal cord injury at birth. The child had some sensation below the level of injury but no functional motor control.

tomic abnormalities obtained from radiographs and CT scans. This bony correction may include a varus osteotomy of the proximal femur or a Pemberton osteotomy for the hip that is dislocating anteriorly. The shelf or Chiari procedures have been less successful in maintaining hip reduction [4]. If the hip is dislocating posteriorly, a Dega osteotomy or a posterior shelf osteotomy as described by Betz and colleagues [15] (Fig. 3) is indicated. Muscle transfers also can be incorporated and, although it is unlikely that this will result in a strong active contraction, a tenodesis effect may result. The authors typically

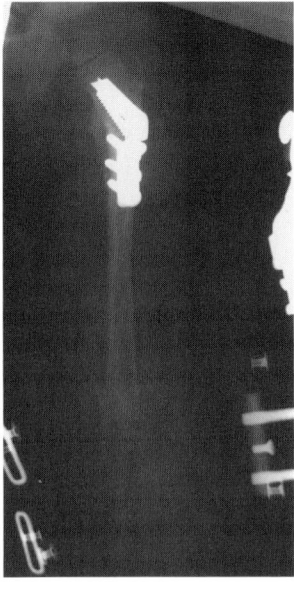

Fig. 6. Distal femur fracture 6 weeks after proximal femoral osteotomy for hip subluxation in a 4-year-old child who had an incomplete T4 SCI.

perform external oblique transfers in children who have flaccid paralysis with functional abdominal musculature. Postoperatively the authors prefer a hip abduction orthosis in an attempt to avoid the skin breakdown issues that often occur with casting. Fig. 4

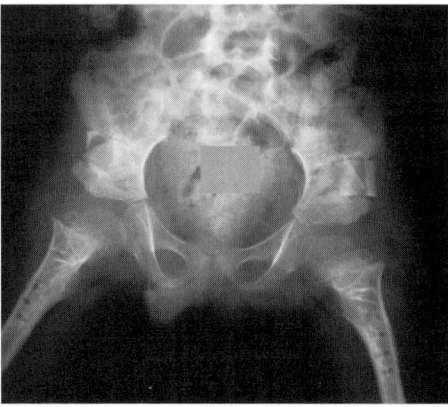

Fig. 5. The same child as in Fig. 4 at age 6 years, 2 years after bilateral pelvic and femoral osteotomies with external oblique transfers to the greater trochanter and subsequent plate removal. The surgery was complicated by a distal femur fracture that occurred 6 weeks after the initial surgery and was treated by immobilization in a splint.

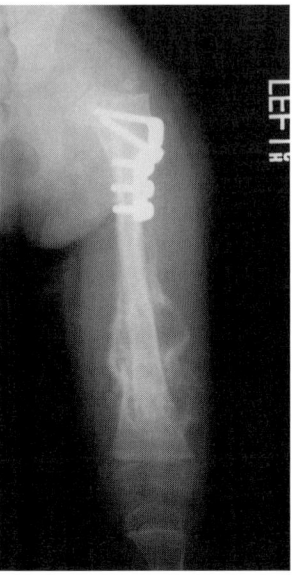

Fig. 7. The same child as in Fig. 6 only 4 weeks after the fracture was diagnosed. Note the exuberant callus formation.

is an AP radiograph of the pelvis of a 4-year-old child with a T4 incomplete spinal cord injury that occurred at birth. They had incomplete sensation below the level of injury but no functional motor control. Fig. 5 is an AP radiograph of the pelvis of the same child at age 6 years, 2 years after bilateral pelvic and femoral osteotomies with external oblique transfers to the greater trochanter and subsequent plate removal. The surgery was complicated by a distal femur fracture that occurred 6 weeks after the initial surgery and was treated by immobilization in a splint (Figs. 6 and 7).

Joint contractures

Contractures are a significant cause of disability in children who have SCI. If not prevented or properly treated, they can lead to problems with standing, sitting tolerance, skin hygiene, ulcerations, joint destruction, and poor self esteem [7,16]. If established early, joint contractures in children cause significant deformities that can be difficult to correct and can lead to bony deformities. The most important aspect of joint contractures is prevention.

The authors strongly encourage families to have their children use nighttime splints for ankle and knee range of motion and to sleep prone to prevent hip flexion contractures. Contractures clearly can prevent upright mobility [7], especially if hip or knee flexion contractures exceed 30°. Unfortunately this occurs in 30% to 50% of children who have SCI [7].

Surgical treatment should be considered for patients for whom conservative care fails or those who desire upright mobility or have other functional deficits believed to be a direct result of the contractures. Often contractures return, especially in the seated population, so that careful assessment of the functional goals and a strong postoperative commitment to therapy (stretching and splinting) is needed before undertaking surgery. The authors avoid casting, especially any attempts at serial casting or wedging, in patients who are insensate.

Treatment of contractures in children who have SCI is different from those who have cerebral palsy. True contractures are much more common, and rarely does tendon lengthening alone provide adequate release. Release of hip flexion contractures usually is performed surgically, and complete release of the hip flexors may be needed. Often a pseudo hip flexion contracture may occur and the fascia overlying the abductors and the tensor fascia (modified Ober-Yount procedure) may need to be released also.

Postoperative prone positioning is critical, as is aggressive physical therapy.

Heterotopic ossification

Unique to children can be the delayed onset of heterotopic ossification (HO). Garland and colleagues [17] showed that pediatric patients can develop HO up to 14 months following injury, whereas adults generally develop it in less than 6 months. They recommend resection of established HO if it is causing blockage in functional joint motion and not to wait until the HO matures. The reason not to wait until the bone matures and the bone scan become quiescent is that there is so much osteopenia in areas such as the femoral neck that the risk for pathologic fractures is too high.

For prophylaxis of HO, one should consider medical treatment of HO at the first sign of radiographic evidence. Prophylactic radiation is strongly recommended in adult patients, but concern regarding the effects of radiation persists in children.

Pathologic fractures

Fractures in children who have SCI occur commonly, with a prevalence of 10% to 20% [18]. Hip fractures are one of the most common injuries, comprising 14% to 47% of pathologic long-bone fractures [19]. Treatment of pathologic long-bone fractures in children who have SCI is typically immobilization with a soft dressing or splinting in an effort to decrease the length of immobilization and prevent skin breakdown from insensate skin beneath the cast [18,20]. Treatment of hip fractures in patients who have SCI is controversial, and there is little literature available on treatment of hip fractures in children who have SCI.

Diagnosis of the fracture can be difficult. One should be aware that this can happen, and during evaluation one should look for deformity, crepitus, swelling, erythema, or systemic fever. Often an initial misdiagnosis of infection is made. If the initial radiographs are negative, the patient should be re-evaluated in 24 hours for clinical signs, with a repeat radiograph and possibly a bone scan.

Complications of fractures include bleeding secondary to femoral fracture, pressure sores secondary to immobilization, autonomic dysreflexia, misdiagnosis of the callus being a malignant tumor, and malalignment. The most important element in preventing a misdiagnosis of callus as an osteosarcoma is to be aware of the radiographic appearance of a pathologic fracture in patients who have paralysis.

The authors reviewed the results of the treatment of hip fractures in children who had SCI. There were seven hip fractures in six patients, five of which were treated surgically. The authors had six complications in seven fractures. These complications included two nonunions of the femoral neck (one in the operative and one in the nonoperative group), two skin ulcers (both from cast treatment), one patient who had heterotopic ossification, and one hardware failure. The hardware failure occurred when a patient who had a femoral neck fracture was treated with two pins that migrated. The authors now use only a sideplate with lag screw and derotational screw. All patients maintained their range of motion from full extension to at least 90° of flexion.

Surgical treatment seemed to have little additional morbidity as compared with immobilization alone. If surgical treatment is undertaken, the authors suggest a sideplate with lag screw and derotational screw. [21] The authors routinely use deep venous thrombosis (DVT) prophylaxis in the form of compression garments and monitor for DVTs with ultrasound evaluation.

The authors recommend a preventive education program for patients that focuses on safety in risk-taking activities, minimizing bone mineral density loss with weightbearing, adequate nutrition, the use of proper equipment for transfers, and attempting to avoid any additional immobilization than normally occurs in children who have SCI.

References

[1] Vogel LC, DeVivo MJ. Etiology and demographics. In: Betz RR, Mulcahey MJ, editors. The child with a spinal cord injury. Rosemont, IL: American Academy of Orthopaedic Surgeons; 1994. p. 3–13.

[2] Stein SC, Feldman JG, Friedlander M, et al. Is myelomeningocele a disappearing disease? Pediatrics 1982; 69:511.

[3] Reimers J. The stability of the hip in children. A radiological study of the results of muscle surgery in cerebral palsy. Acta Orthop Scand Suppl 1980;184:1–100.

[4] McCarthy JJ, Weibel B, Betz RR. Results of pelvic osteotomies for hip subluxation or dislocation in children with spinal cord injury. Topics SCI Rehab 2000;6S:48–53.

[5] McCarthy JJ, Chafetz RS, Betz RR, et al. The incidence and degree of hip subluxation/dislocation in children with spinal cord injury. J Spinal Cord Med 2004;27(Suppl 1):S80–3.

[6] Rink P, Miller F. Hip instability in spinal cord injury patients. J Pediatr Orthop 1990;10:583–7.

[7] Vogel LC, Lubicky JP. Ambulation in children and adolescents with spinal cord injuries. J Pediatr Orthop 1995;15:501–16.

[8] Betz RR. Unique management needs of pediatric spinal cord injury patients: orthopaedic problems in the child with spinal cord injury. J Spinal Cord Med 1997;20: 14–6.

[9] Vogel LC, Krajci KA, Anderson CJ. Adults with pediatric-onset spinal cord injury, part 2: musculoskeletal and neurological complications. J Spinal Cord Med 2002;25:117–23.

[10] Vogel LC, Gogia RS, Lubicky JP. Hip abnormalities in children with spinal cord injury [abstract]. J Spinal Cord Med 1995;18:172.

[11] Pierre-Jacques H, Betz RR, Berman AT, et al. Hip instability in children with spinal cord injuries. American Academy of Orthopaedic Surgeons Annual Meeting, Orlando, Florida, February 16–21, 1995.

[12] Han M, Kim H. Chronic hip instability as a cause of autonomic dysreflexia: successful management by resection arthroplasty: a case report. J Bone Joint Surg [Am] 2003;85:126–8.

[13] Baird RA, DeBenedetti MJ, Eltorai I. Non-septic hip instability in the chronic spinal cord injury patient. Paraplegia 1986;24:293–300.

[14] Bonaroti D, Akers JM, Smith BT, et al. Comparison of functional electrical stimulation to long leg braces for upright mobility in children with complete thoracic level spinal injuries. Arch Phys Med Rehabil 1999; 80:1047–53.

[15] Betz RR, Mulcahey MJ, Smith BT, et al. Implications of hip subluxation for FES-assisted mobility in patients with spinal cord injury. Orthopedics 2001;24:181–4.

[16] Dalyan M, Sherman A, Cardenas DD. Factors associated with contractures in acute spinal cord injury. Spinal Cord 1998;36:405–8.

[17] Garland DE, Shimoyama ST, Lugo C, et al. Spinal cord insults and heterotopic ossification in the pediatric population. Clin Orthop 1989;245:303–10.

[18] Betz RR, Mulcahey MJ. Spinal cord injury rehabilitation. In: Weinstein SL, editor. The pediatric spine: principles and practice. New York: Raven Press, Ltd.; 1994. p. 781–810.

[19] Freehafer AA, Mast WA. Lower extremity fractures in patients with spinal-cord injury. J Bone Joint Surg Am 1965;47(4):683–94.

[20] Eichenholtz SN. Management of long-bone fractures in paraplegic patients. J Bone Joint Surg Am 1963; 45(2):299–310.

[21] McCarthy JJ, Betz RR. The treatment of hip fractures in children with existing spinal cord injuries. Top SCI Rehab 2000;6S:42–7.

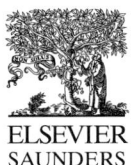

Evaluation and Treatment of Hip Dysplasia in Charcot-Marie-Tooth Disease

Gilbert Chan, MD[a], J. Richard Bowen, MD[a], S. Jay Kumar, MD[a,b],*

[a]Department of Orthopedics, Alfred I. duPont Hospital for Children, 1600 Rockland Road, Wilmington, DE 19803, USA
[b]Thomas Jefferson University, 1020 Walnut Street, Philadelphia, PA 19107, USA

Charcot-Marie-Tooth disease (CMTD), also known as hereditary motor and sensory neuropathy, is the most common form of heritable peripheral neuropathy [1] with a prevalence of 1 in 2500 children [2,3]. The disorder has been divided into two groups: type 1 and type 2 [4]. CMTD type 1, which is the demyelinating form of the disease, is more common, affecting approximately 60% to 80% of the general CMTD population; CMTD type 2, the axonal form of the disorder, affects 20% to 40% of the general CMTD population [5]. For both types, the most common form of inheritance is an autosomal dominant pattern, although autosomal recessive, X chromosome-linked, and sporadic transmission have been reported [5]. A general comparison of the types is shown in Table 1.

The most common genetic defect seen in CMTD has been linked to chromosome 17p11.2 and is caused by a duplication of the PMP22 gene. This particular defect affects approximately 70% of families that have type 1 CMTD; it is also the most common cause of sporadic mutation and accounts for 52% of all cases of CMTD [6–8]. Numerous other genetic mutations have been identified and implicated to cause the various types/subtypes of CMTD, which may account for the variability in presentation and severity of involvement.

CMTD is a chronic progressive peripheral neuropathy. The onset of the disease is slow and insidious.

CMTD types 1 and 2 are similar phenotypically and are difficult to distinguish clinically. In general CMTD manifests with distal weakness, affecting the intrinsic and the extrinsic musculature of the extremities [9–11]. Sensory deficits and areflexia may also occur. Muscle weakness leads to an imbalance resulting in the deformities characteristic of the disease.

Most patients present with cavovarus or "high-arched feet," which typically is the hallmark of the disorder. This condition is often bilateral and patients complain of difficulty in shoe wear, painful calluses under the base of the fifth metatarsal, metatarsal heads and heel, and pain with prolonged standing or activity. The associated claw toe deformity makes shoe wear difficult, and patients have pain over the dorsal aspect of the toes where the shoe rubs over the prominent interphalangeal joints. Other orthopedic concerns include an abnormal gait pattern, which is because of weak ankle dorsiflexors causing footdrop. The pelvis compensates for this inability to dorsiflex the ankle by raising the pelvis to provide clearance, producing a "marionette gait" pattern [11]. The prevalence of scoliosis is similar to that of idiopathic scoliosis [12,13].

Hip abnormalities were not appreciated until recently. The association of hip dysplasia and CMTD was first reported by Kumar and colleagues [14]. Since then, there have been numerous reports in the literature associating hip dysplasia with CMTD [15–21]. The initial report by Kumar and colleagues increased awareness of the association of hip dysplasia with CMTD. The general prevalence of hip dysplasia in CMTD is not clear. Walker and colleagues [21] reviewed 74 radiographs and found a total of 6 dysplastic hips (8.1%). They also reported

* Corresponding author. Department of Orthopedics, Alfred I. duPont Hospital for Children, 1600 Rockland Road., Wilmington, DE 19803.
E-mail address: sjayakum@nemours.org (S.J. Kumar).

Table 1
Comparison of Charcot-Marie-Tooth disease, types 1 and 2

	CMTD 1	CMTD 2
Description	Myelinopathy	Axonopathy
Pattern of inheritance	AD[a], AR, X-linked, sporadic	AD[a], AR, X-linked, sporadic
Electrophysiologic findings	<38 m/sec	Normal to slightly decreased
Pathologic findings	Segmental demyelination/remyelination, onion bulb appearance	Axonal loss, absent to few onion bulbs
Age at onset	Early first to second decade of life	Second decade of life, may occur later

Abbreviations: AD, autosomal dominant; AR, autosomal recessive; CMTD, Charcot-Marie-Tooth disease; m, meter; sec, second; X, X chromosome.

[a] The most common pattern of inheritance.

hip abnormalities in 21 of 74 patients (35%). Their criteria for diagnosing hip dysplasia were a neck-shaft angle of greater than 147°, center-edge angle of less than 20°, and a Reimer's migration percentage of greater than or equal to 20% [21]. Hip dysplasia is a serious condition, which may be congenital, developmental, or neuromuscular in origin. If left untreated, the hip abnormalities may lead to pain and gait abnormalities. Therefore, early recognition and appropriate treatment of this condition is essential to avoid future morbidity.

Hip dysplasia in Charcot-Marie-Tooth disease

The hips in patients who have CMTD are normal at birth. When the hips are abnormal or dysplastic at birth, it is probably congenital in nature and should

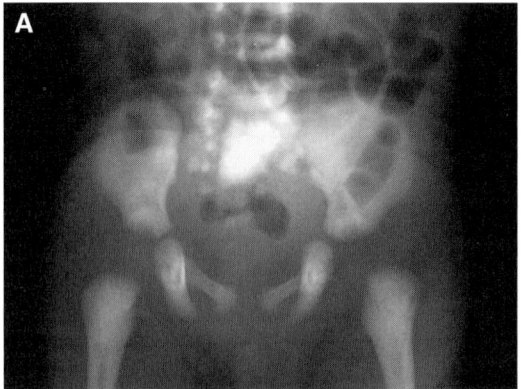
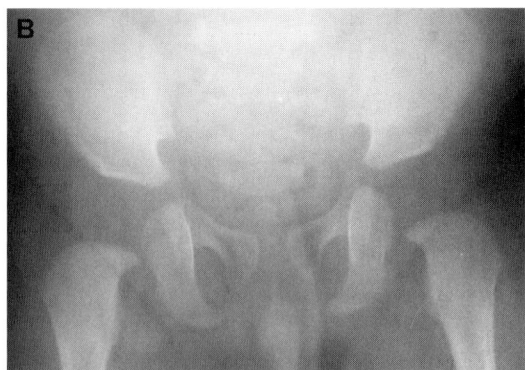
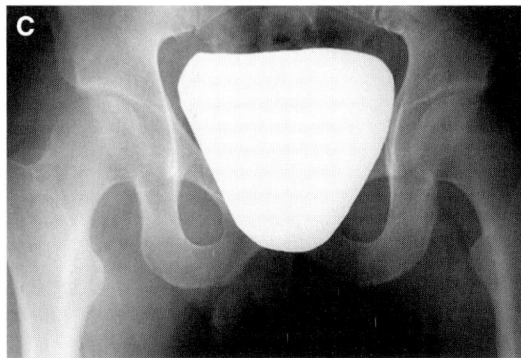

Fig. 1. (*A*) Antero-posterior radiograph of the pelvis in an infant diagnosed with developmental dysplasia of the hip. He was treated with a Pavlik harness. (*B*) Radiograph taken one month after removal of the Pavlik harness shows well-reduced hips. (*C*) Radiograph taken at 32 years follow-up shows normal hips.

be managed as a case of developmental dysplasia of the hip (DDH). There is no reason why a patient diagnosed with CMTD later on in life could not have DDH at birth. This DDH has to be recognized and treated appropriately (Fig. 1).

Hip abnormalities in CMTD are not easily recognized. While routine screening with standing anteroposterior radiographs of all patients with CMTD is necessary, any patient who has a Trendelenburg gait (a waddling gait caused by paralysis of the gluteal muscles) or sway while walking should have the hips examined carefully. The hip disorder in CMTD is neuromuscular in origin. The origin of this process in the hip may be divided into two parts, the primary deforming force and the secondary deformity. The primary deforming force is weakness of the proximal musculature of the hip, predominantly the hip abductors and extensors, that over time cause a shallow acetabulum and a valgus anteverted femoral neck.

The clinical presentation and the age at presentation of these hips can be variable, which is reflective of the same variability in severity found in the disease. In the authors' experience, the more severely involved patient will tend to present with hip problems earlier. Initially, most patients do not present with any complaints and may remain asymptomatic for a prolonged period of time. Still others are found as incidental findings from radiographs taken for other reasons or from screening close relatives presenting with similar problems. This fact may mask the overall prevalence of the disease, and many patients may go undetected for years. Others present as gait abnormalities. The presence of pain is a later manifestation of the disease, which may indicate marked subluxation and arthrosis of the joint [18]. In the absence of intracranial or spine pathology, an eight- or nine-year-old child presenting with primary acetabular dysplasia and a valgus anteverted femoral neck should be evaluated for CMTD.

Evaluation

A standard evaluation of a child who has CMTD begins with a detailed examination, which includes a family history and physical examination. Clinical symptoms combined with a positive family history lead to a high index of suspicion for the presence of CMTD. Electrophysiologic testing (electromyogram/nerve conduction velocity [EMG/NCV]) or DNA analy-

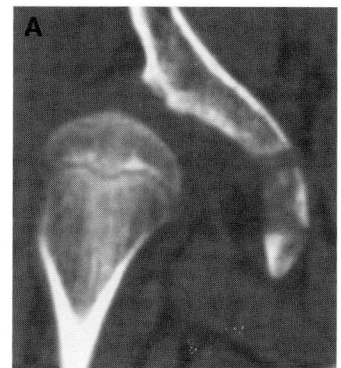
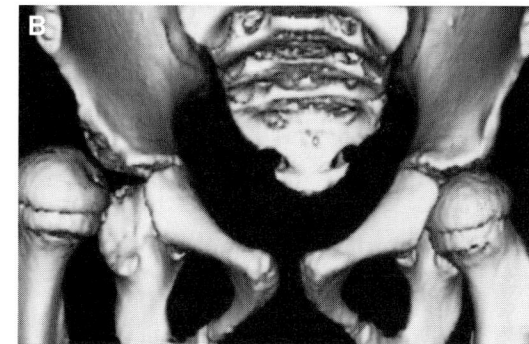
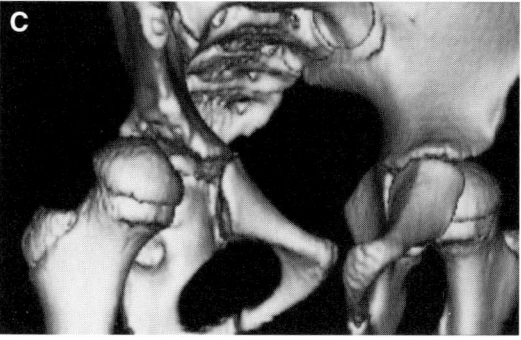

Fig. 2. (*A*) CT scan showing acetabular dysplasia and a subluxated femoral head. (*B*) Anteroposterior and (*C*) oblique three dimensional reconstructions showing the acetabular deficiency and the proximal femoral dysplasia.

sis can confirm the diagnosis and help in distinguishing the various types or subtypes [5]. Sural nerve biopsy may also be used to confirm the diagnosis; however, the pain and morbidity that may be associated with the procedure do not make it a favored choice [22–24]. The EMG/NCV findings associated with type 1 CMTD show a slow conduction velocity (<38 m/sec), which is normal or slightly prolonged in type 2. DNA analysis is currently being used and is accurate for the more common genotypes involved; however, a negative result does not rule out the presence of any of the various subtypes of the disorder because of the wide variety of genetic mutations seen.

Once the diagnosis of CMTD is established, a standing antero-posterior radiograph of the pelvis should be performed. Because the natural history of hip dysplasia in patients who have CMTD is not known, if the hips are found to be normal, follow-up radiographs at least once every 2 years should be performed. An infant of a patient known to have CMTD should have a screening ultrasound of the hips. On the other hand, if dysplasia is documented, a thorough evaluation of the hip should be done. The amount of acetabular dysplasia, the center-edge angle, femoral-head coverage, femoral neck valgus and degree of migration or subluxation of the femoral head, femoral anteversion, and degenerative changes should be noted. A supine pelvic radiograph with the femur in 20° to 30° of abduction and 20° to 30° of internal rotation will help determine the true amount of femoral neck valgus and the amount of femoral anteversion present. The radiographic findings should be correlated with the clinical findings to plan proper treatment.

A CT scan, particularly a three-dimensional reconstruction, may be helpful in quantitative analysis of acetabular dysplasia (Fig. 2). The CT scan may also be useful in identifying any rotational deformities of the femur. An ultrasound may be useful if hip laxity is noted at birth; however, this condition is DDH and should be treated as such. Other imaging modalities have little to no role in evaluation of hip disease in CMTD.

Treatment

Hip dysplasia in CMTD requires treatment, even when the hip is asymptomatic. Nonsurgical modalities of treatment, such as braces, have no role in

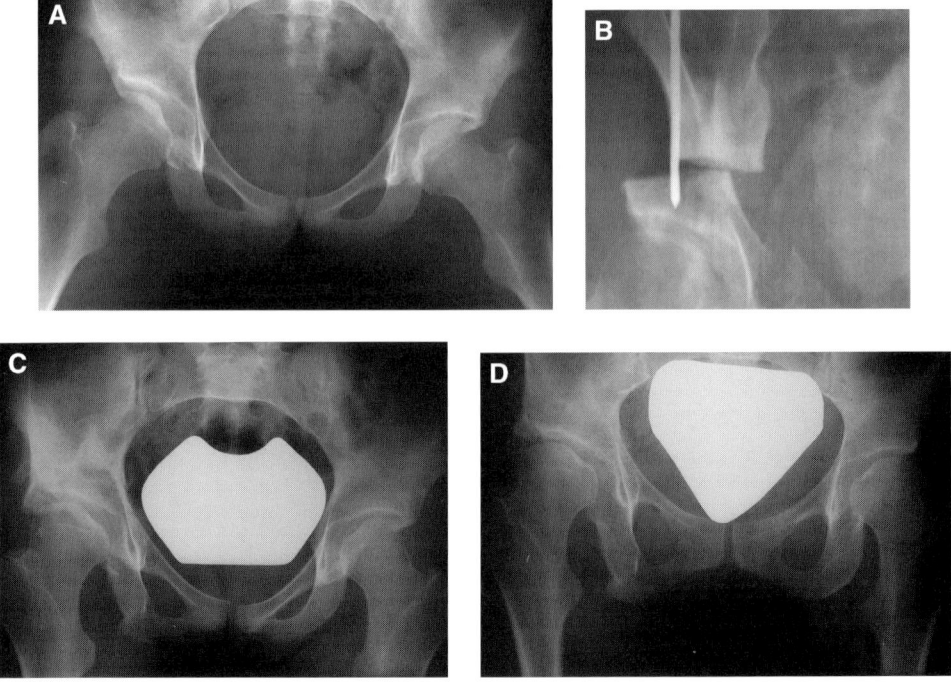

Fig. 3. (*A*) 15-year-old child diagnosed with type 1 CMTD who has dysplasia of the right hip. (*B*) She underwent a triple osteotomy of the hip. (*C*) Results showing good coverage, obviating the need for a proximal femoral procedure. (*D*) Follow-up at 29 years of age showing adequate coverage.

treating these hips. Physical therapy may have a role in maintaining range of motion and strengthening hip abductors and extensors. Almost all studies recommend operative reconstruction as the treatment of choice [14,15,17,18,20].

Even though the pathology of hip dysplasia has an acetabular and proximal femoral component, it is better to address the acetabular deficiency first (Fig. 3). Children who have weak hip abductors do not function well after a femoral varus osteotomy and their Trendelenburg gait tends to worsen. Hence, it is better to address the acetabular dysplasia first; and if dysplasia and subluxation persist, then a proximal femoral varus derotation osteotomy with rigid internal fixation should be performed. A wide variety of pelvic osteotomies have been described in the literature to address this problem. Among these are the Salter [14], Salter with a concomitant shelf procedure [17], periacetabular osteotomy [25], triple osteotomy [20], and the Chiari osteotomy [21,26].

A factor to consider in treating these hips is the sensitivity of the nerves to stretch. Most of the innominate osteotomies are opening wedge osteotomies that lengthen the innominate bone and are likely to stretch the sciatic nerve. Kumar and colleagues [14] reported two children treated with a Salter innominate osteotomy. Of these, one child developed sciatic nerve palsy postoperatively. Van Erve and Dreissen [20] reported the development of peroneal nerve palsy secondary to compression of the nerve in the traction mattress. Care should be taken when performing the acetabular procedure so as not to apply undue stretch on the nerve or cause direct injury by retractors in the sciatic notch. Currently, the authors prefer to perform a modification of the triple osteotomy as described by Lipton and Bowen [27], which is a closing wedge osteotomy (Fig. 4). The use of intraoperative monitoring by somatosensory-evoked potentials and motor-evoked potentials while performing the procedures may help prevent irreversible damage to the nerve.

Once the acetabular deficiency is corrected, the femoral component of the hip dysplasia may need to be assessed. The hip should be taken through its full range of motion to assess for adequacy of coverage, proper seating of the femoral head within the hip

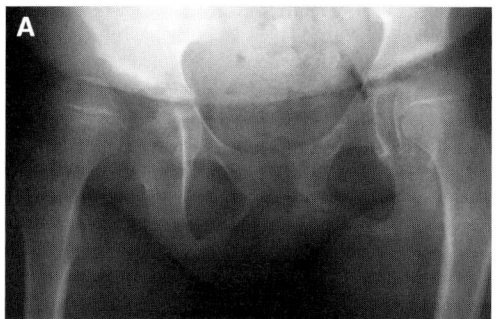
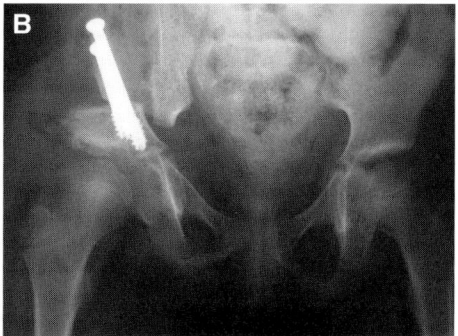
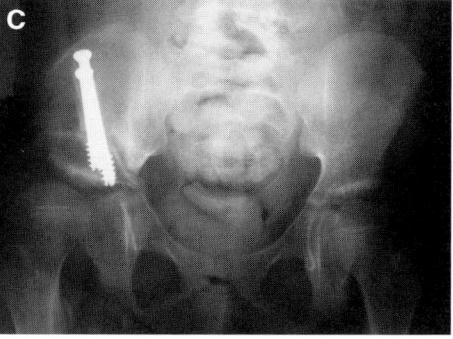

Fig. 4. (*A*) A 9-year-old child who has acetabular dysplasia, subluxation of the femoral head, and increased valgus of the femoral neck. (*B*) She underwent triple innominate osteotomy as modified by Bowen and Lipton, which was able to address the acetabular dysplasia. (*C*) On follow-up the femoral neck valgus and anteversion resulted in lateralization of the femoral head, which will be addressed with a proximal femoral osteotomy.

joint, and any signs of impingement or subluxation. If there is any doubt, an intraoperative arthrogram may help identify signs of impingement as well as check for coverage.

If after the pelvic reconstruction all the components of the dysplasia are not corrected, then the deformity in the proximal femur should be addressed. If the problem is secondary to anteversion, a derotation should be performed. If there is increased femoral neck valgus, a varus osteotomy will be needed. Care should be taken when performing the varus osteotomy because excessive varus might further weaken the already-compromised hip abductors. The femoral osteotomy should be rigidly fixed with internal fixation, and spica casts should be avoided because their use can further weaken the muscles around the hip.

Summary

Hip dysplasia in CMTD results from the weakness of the hip abductors and extensors, which produces abnormal joint mechanics leading to a shallow acetabulum with changes in the proximal femur. Clinical presentation is variable and may depend on the severity of the disease. Initially most hips are asymptomatic, but may become painful secondary to subluxation and degenerative changes. Acetabular reconstruction should be performed initially, followed by femoral reconstruction if acetabular reconstruction alone does not correct the hip dysplasia. Early ambulation following surgery is mandatory in these children.

References

[1] Skre H. Genetic and clinical aspects of Charcot-Marie-Tooth's disease. Clin Genet 1974;6(2):98–118.
[2] Emery AE. Population frequencies of inherited neuromuscular diseases–a world survey. Neuromuscul Disord 1991;1(1):19–29.
[3] Lupski JR, Wise CA, Kuwano A, et al. Gene dosage is a mechanism for Charcot-Marie-Tooth disease type 1A. Nat Genet 1992;1(1):29–33.
[4] Dyck PJ, Lambert EH. Lower motor and primary sensory neuron diseases with peroneal muscular atrophy. I. Neurologic, genetic, and electrophysiologic findings in hereditary polyneuropathies. Arch Neurol 1968;18(6):603–18.
[5] Saifi GM, Szigeti K, Snipes GJ, et al. Molecular mechanisms, diagnosis, and rational approaches to management of and therapy for Charcot-Marie-Tooth disease and related peripheral neuropathies. J Investig Med 2003;51(5):261–83.
[6] Hoogendijk JE, Hensels GW, Gabreels-Festen AA, et al. De-novo mutation in hereditary motor and sensory neuropathy type I. Lancet 1992;339(8801):1081–2.
[7] Nelis E, Van Broeckhoven C, De Jonghe P, et al. Estimation of the mutation frequencies in Charcot-Marie-Tooth disease type 1 and hereditary neuropathy with liability to pressure palsies: a European collaborative study. Eur J Hum Genet 1996;4(1):25–33.
[8] Wise CA, Garcia CA, Davis SN, et al. Molecular analyses of unrelated Charcot-Marie-Tooth (CMT) disease patients suggest a high frequency of the CMT1A duplication. Am J Hum Genet 1993;53(4):853–63.
[9] Mann RA, Missirian J. Pathophysiology of Charcot-Marie-Tooth disease. Clin Orthop 1988;234:221–8.
[10] Sabir M, Lyttle D. Pathogenesis of pes cavus in Charcot-Marie-Tooth disease. Clin Orthop 1983;175:173–8.
[11] Sabir M, Lyttle D. Pathogenesis of Charcot-Marie-Tooth disease. Gait analysis and electrophysiologic, genetic, histopathologic, and enzyme studies in a kinship. Clin Orthop 1984;184:223–35.
[12] Daher YH, Lonstein JE, Winter RB, et al. Spinal deformities in patients with Charcot-Marie-tooth disease. A review of 12 patients. Clin Orthop 1986;202:219–22.
[13] Hensinger RN, MacEwen GD. Spinal deformity associated with heritable neurological conditions: spinal muscular atrophy, Friedreich's ataxia, familial dysautonomia, and Charcot-Marie-Tooth disease. J Bone Joint Surg Am 1976;58(1):13–24.
[14] Kumar SJ, Marks HG, Bowen JR, et al. Hip dysplasia associated with Charcot-Marie-Tooth disease in the older child and adolescent. J Pediatr Orthop 1985;5(5):511–4.
[15] Cucuzzella TR, Guille JT, MacEwen GD. Charcot-Marie-Tooth disease associated with hip dysplasia: a case report. Del Med J 1996;68(6):305–7.
[16] Fuller JE, DeLuca PA. Acetabular dysplasia and Charcot-Marie-Tooth disease in a family. A report of four cases. J Bone Joint Surg Am 1995;77(7):1087–91.
[17] McGann R, Gurd A. The association between Charcot-Marie-Tooth disease and developmental dysplasia of the hip. Orthopedics 2002;25(3):337–9.
[18] Pailthorpe CA, Benson MK. Hip dysplasia in hereditary motor and sensory neuropathies. J Bone Joint Surg Br 1992;74(4):538–40.
[19] Ushiyama T, Tanaka C, Kawasaki T, et al. Hip dysplasia in Charcot-Marie-Tooth disease: report of a family. J Orthop Sci 2003;8(4):610–2.
[20] van Erve RH, Driessen AP. Developmental hip dysplasia in hereditary motor and sensory neuropathy type 1. J Pediatr Orthop 1999;19(1):92–6.
[21] Walker JL, Nelson KR, Heavilon JA, et al. Hip abnormalities in children with Charcot-Marie-Tooth disease. J Pediatr Orthop 1994;14(1):54–9.
[22] Brunelli GA. Prevention of damage caused by sural nerve withdrawal for nerve grafting. Hand Surg 2002;7(2):163–6.
[23] Poburski R, Malin JP, Stark E. Sequelae of sural nerve biopsies. Clin Neurol Neurosurg 1985;87(3):193–8.

[24] Schoeller T, Huemer GM, Shafighi M, et al. Microsurgical repair of the sural nerve after nerve biopsy to avoid associated sensory morbidity: a preliminary report. Neurosurgery 2004;54(4):897–900 [discussion 900–1].

[25] Trumble SJ, Mayo KA, Mast JW. The periacetabular osteotomy. Minimum 2 year followup in more than 100 hips. Clin Orthop 1999;363:54–63.

[26] Osebold WR, Lester EL, Watson P. Dynamics of hip joint remodeling after Chiari osteotomy. 10 patients with neuromuscular disease followed for 8 years. Acta Orthop Scand 1997;68(2):128–32.

[27] Lipton GE, Bowen JR. A new modified technique of triple osteotomy of the innominate bone for acetabular dysplasia. Clin Orthop 2005;434:78–85.

Controversies in Slipped Capital Femoral Epiphysis

Randall T. Loder, MD[a,b,*]

[a]Pediatric Orthopaedic Surgery, Indiana University School of Medicine, 541 Clinical Drive, Suite 600, Indianapolis IN 46202, USA
[b]Pediatric Orthopaedics, James Whitcomb Riley Hospital for Children, Room 4250, 702 Barnhill Drive, Indianapolis, IN 46202, USA

Slipped capital femoral epiphysis (SCFE) is a common adolescent hip disorder. This article reviews the major controversies in SCFE as of the year 2005. These are (1) treatment of the unstable SCFE, (2) the role of osteotomy in the treatment of SCFE, (3) prophylactic fixation of the contralateral hip in children presenting with unilateral SCFE, and (4) methods of fixation in the very young child with SCFE.

Treatment of the unstable slipped capital femoral epiphysis

The traditional classification for an SCFE has been acute, chronic, and acute-on-chronic [1,2]. The differentiation between these three types was mostly temporal; an acute SCFE had symptoms for <3 weeks, a chronic SCFE for >3 weeks, and an acute-on-chronic SCFE for >3 weeks with a recent exacerbation of symptoms. This classification can be inaccurate because of the inability of parents and children to remember exactly when symptoms began and because of the prognosis of the SCFE. In 1993 new classifications dependent on the stability of the SCFE were described [3,4] in an attempt to impart prognosis. It makes sense that an unstable SCFE is more likely to experience complications than a stable SCFE, in whatever way stability is defined. The most significant complication with an unstable SCFE is avascular necrosis (AVN). The development of AVN in a child who has SCFE nearly always results in degenerative hip disease later in life, albeit at different ages and rates of joint deterioration [5–7]. Stability thus imparts prognosis.

Stability is defined clinically using the ability to walk. A stable SCFE is when the child can walk with or without crutches; an unstable SCFE is when the child cannot walk with or without crutches [4]. The prognosis for a child who has a stable SCFE is very good, with a prevalence of AVN approaching zero [4,8]. The prognosis for a child who has an unstable SCFE is guarded because of the increased risk for AVN; the prevalence of AVN ranges from 3% to 84% [1,4,7–12]. Approximately 5% of SCFEs are unstable. Most unstable SCFEs present as a unilateral SCFE or as a sequential second SCFE of a patient who has a previous unilateral stable SCFE. Bilateral unstable SCFEs are extremely rare. Because only 5% of all unstable SCFEs are bilateral [11], only 0.25% of all children who have SCFE have bilateral unstable SCFEs ([0.05][0.05] = 0.0025).

Children who have unstable SCFEs present with extreme hip and thigh pain [4,11,13]. A history of trauma, eg, a trip off the curb, a fall in sports, or other mild traumatic event, is frequently present. The child lies perfectly still with the lower extremity in a position of flexion, abduction, and external rotation. Any attempts to move the lower extremity actively or passively are resisted. The presentation is similar to that of a displaced femoral neck fracture, and in es-

---

This work was supported in part by the Garceau Professorship Endowment, Department of Orthopaedic Surgery, Indiana University School of Medicine, and the Rapp Pediatric Orthopaedic Research Fund, Riley Children's Foundation.

* Pediatric Orthopaedics, James Whitcomb Riley Hospital for Children, Room 4250, 702 Barnhill Drive, Indianapolis, IN 46202.
E-mail address: rloder@iupui.edu

sence it is a displaced Salter–Harris I fracture of the proximal femoral physis, which explains the painful nature and high AVN rate. Because of this clinical presentation unstable SCFEs have been termed fracturelike SCFEs by some investigators [13].

In an unstable SCFE an AP pelvis radiograph is often the only view that can be obtained because of the child's discomfort. The diagnosis is readily made, as the AP radiograph demonstrates an abrupt displacement of the epiphysis on the metaphysis (Fig. 1); if the SCFE is acute-on-chronic using the older classification scheme, then variable degrees of metaphyseal remodeling along the superior and anterior femoral neck are seen [1,2,4]. If it is an acute type using the older classification scheme, remodeling of the superior and anterior femoral neck are not visualized (Fig. 1). Once the unstable SCFE has been diagnosed on the AP radiograph, and if the patient permits, a true or cross-table lateral radiograph should be taken. A frog-lateral radiograph should not be attempted because of significant discomfort and the risk for further iatrogenic slipping. If a lateral radiograph can be obtained and anterior physeal separation is noted, then the risk for AVN is increased [14]. A frog-lateral or cross-table lateral view of the opposite hip also should be obtained; it is easy to forget this in the excitement of assessing the unstable side.

Treatment of an unstable SCFE is controversial. It must be clearly stated that the best method for treatment of an unstable SCFE is still controversial and there are no good data supporting one approach over another. The goals of treatment are to (1) prevent further slipping until physeal closure, (2) avoid complications, primarily those of AVN, and (3) maintain adequate hip function [15]. Possible treatment options for unstable SCFEs are (1) internal fixation, (2) epiphysiodesis, (3) proximal femoral osteotomy, and (4) surgical dislocation of the hip with open reduction, femoral osteotomy, and fixation of the SCFE. Adequate preoperative AP and lateral radiographs of both hips are needed. This is to ensure that a contralateral SCFE is not missed. If an undiagnosed SCFE is present on the opposite side, increased physeal shear stress is placed on the opposite hip after operative treatment of the unstable SCFE. This can

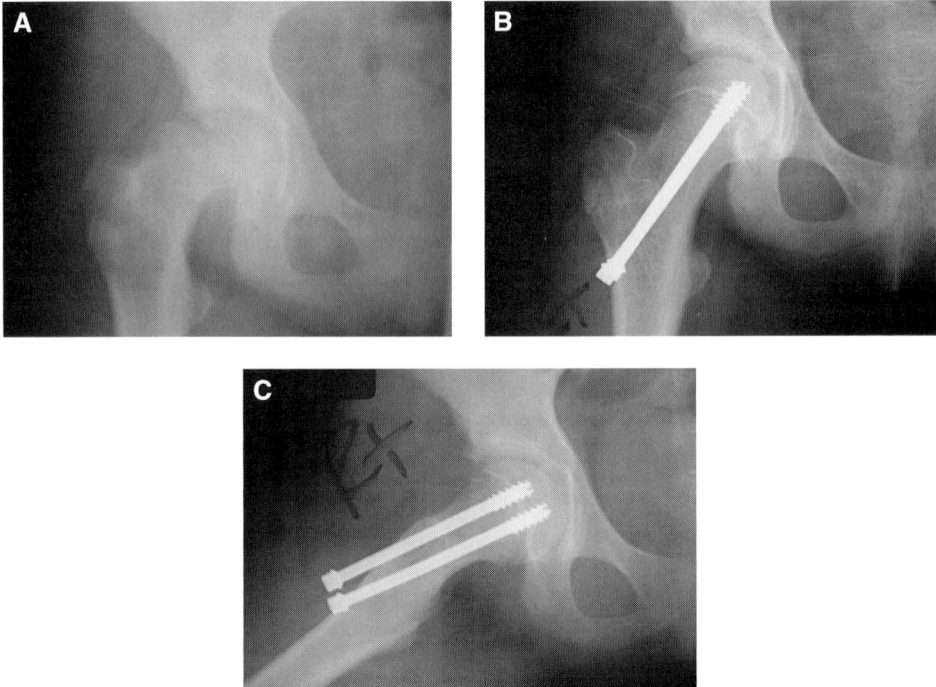

Fig. 1. A 13-year, 6-month-old girl with an unstable SCFE. (*A*) The AP radiograph at presentation. Note the abrupt displacement of the epiphysis on the metaphysis. No lateral radiograph was obtainable. (*B*) The AP and (*C*) lateral radiographs after gentle repositioning and internal fixation with two cannulated screws. Note that there is no early remodeling of the femoral metaphysis indicating the sudden onset of the SCFE without any underlying pre-existing stable SCFE component.

result in progression of the undiagnosed SCFE, or worse, convert a stable SCFE to an unstable one.

Although many investigators recommend internal fixation of an unstable SCFE, there is controversy in the timing of fixation, the role of preoperative traction, the role of reduction and decompression, and the number of screws used for fixation [16]. Gordon and colleagues [17] described 16 consecutive unstable SCFEs, with 2 developing AVN. Ten children were treated within 24 hours of the onset of acute symptoms with reduction (open or closed), fixation with two cannulated screws, and formal arthrotomy or percutaneous capsulotomy for joint decompression. In these 10 children none (0%) developed AVN. Of the remaining six children (33%), treatment occurred >24 hours after onset of acute symptoms or did not involve joint decompression; two of the six children (33%) developed AVN. They thus recommend early reduction of unstable SCFE with arthrotomy and two cannulated screw fixation to minimize the risk for AVN. The number of SCFEs in their series is small, however. Their recommendations are supported by the angiographic studies of Maeda and colleagues [18] in five unstable SCFEs. In three of the five unstable SCFEs, the superior retinacular vessels did not demonstrate any blood flow. In one case, angiography was performed before and after reduction of the unstable SCFE. In that case, there was no blood flow to the capital epiphysis before reduction, which returned with reduction. They concluded that the vascular injury in unstable SCFE occurs at the time of injury, and that gentle reduction in and of itself does not necessarily contribute to the risk for AVN. Other clinical studies support this belief [11,19].

With these recent studies in mind, the author's personal approach to the treatment of a child who has an unstable SCFE is to proceed immediately with a gentle repositioning, two-screw fixation, and mini-arthrotomy for joint decompression. The child is transferred gently from the bed and positioned on the fracture table after induction of anesthesia. The limb is placed gently in a position of neutral rotation without longitudinal traction if there has been no pre-existing chronic SCFE. The induction of anesthesia removes the child's muscle spasm and guarding. This often results in a spontaneous, unintentional reduction of the slip with simple positioning of the child on the fracture table. This unintentional reduction does not seem to increase the risk for AVN [8,9,11], although one series suggests otherwise [12]. Excessive internal rotation or longitudinal traction is not used, and the author does not use any intentional reduction maneuver unless the deformity is so severe that adequate internal fixation is not possible because of inadequate osseous contact between the epiphysis and metaphysis. If manipulative reduction is necessary, it should be performed only to the chronic position or the position needed to allow adequate osseous contact for stable, adequate screw fixation [10,20].

Cannulated screw fixation then proceeds in the usual fashion. The first screw should be placed in the center of the epiphysis in AP and lateral planes, exactly as with a stable SCFE. The use of a second screw is controversial. A second screw controls rotation and increases stability. Biomechanical studies, however, do not show a twofold increase in strength with two screws, and any screw off the center axis has a much higher chance of joint penetration [21,22]. If a second screw is used, it therefore should be placed inferior to the first screw and with the final tip position at least 1 cm from the subchondral bone to reduce the risk for intra-articular penetration. Postoperatively the child is allowed to get up with crutches once comfortable [23,24]. If there is any question regarding compliance or stability of fixation, the use of a wheelchair for the first 6 weeks is recommended. Nonweightbearing is maintained until early callus is seen along the posterior–inferior metaphysis. Once there is evidence of early healing, gradual and progressive weightbearing is allowed. This typically begins at 8 to 12 weeks. Progression to full weightbearing is usually achieved 3 to 4 months after fixation. Close follow-up to observe for the potential development of AVN is mandatory; AVN usually occurs within the first 12 months after the slip.

Several recent series have recommended in situ fixation with a single central cannulated screw rather than any gentle repositioning with two cannulated screws [12,16]. In the past, bedrest for 1 or 2 weeks before surgery had been recommend; this allowed the joint to quiet down, early healing to occur, and a more stable situation to develop [23]. How this approach affects an acute disruption in epiphyseal blood supply is unknown. If surgery is not performed immediately, but within a few days, the question of preoperative traction (skin or skeletal) arises [13]. The proponents of gentle preoperative traction argue that it allows for a gradual reduction in the hopes of reducing the risk for AVN. This approach only works by reducing any component of AVN that would be caused by an immediate reduction when the slip itself has not resulted in compromised epiphyseal vascularity. Extension decreases intracapsular volume, makes the child more uncomfortable, and theoretically increases the risk for AVN.

Another treatment option is bone graft epiphysiodesis (Schmidt technique) [25]. This percutaneous allograft epiphysiodesis is analogous to in situ fixation using a single central screw [25]. Stability of the SCFE is determined radiographically on the fracture table by gently moving the hip under the image intensifier. If the epiphysis moves relative to the metaphysis, the slip is considered unstable. A guide pin entry point is determined as for an in situ single screw fixation. After the pin has crossed the physis, the tip is advanced to the proper depth, stopping within 2 mm of the subchondral bone but not penetrating the joint. A second guide pin is placed parallel to the first, which secures the femoral epiphysis during subsequent reaming. The femoral neck is reamed to a depth of ~10 mm beyond the physis. A cortical strut allograft is fashioned to the appropriate dimensions and passed over the guide pin and across the physis at least 1 cm. A spica cast is used for 6 to 8 weeks. After cast removal, continued nonweightbearing until physeal closure is recommended. Full weightbearing is usually achieved 10 weeks after surgery [25,26].

Because AVN (Fig. 2) is the most frequent serious complication with an unstable SCFE, are there predictive risk factors? Many potential risk factors have been described (Table 1). These include gender and race of the child, slip magnitude, preoperative traction, the role of reduction, fixation with one or two screws, and timing of surgical fixation/reduction [23,24]. If an unstable SCFE is like a displaced femoral neck fracture in a young adult regarding AVN, then an immediate anatomic reduction should be obtained (closed or open if necessary), and the hip joint decompressed to relieve intracapsular pressure, all in the hopes of reducing the risk for AVN. The present data, however, are conflicting regarding this approach. One question is the role of reduction. Does it correlate with AVN? This is controversial. Some series note that the occurrence or magnitude of reduction does not correlate with the development of AVN [9–11,27], although others come to the opposite conclusion [7,12]. Another question is the timing of reduction. Is an early reduction correlated with a reduced AVN rate? In some series there was no demonstration of an early reduction reducing the

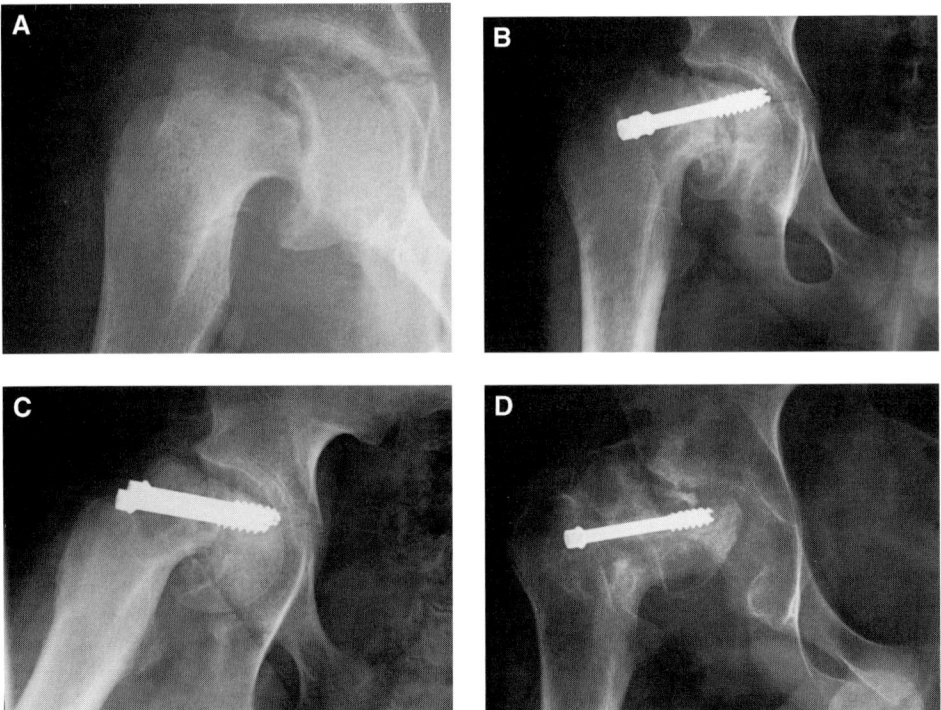

Fig. 2. (*A*) A radiograph of a 12-year-old boy with an unstable SCFE. Note the marked and abrupt displacement of the epiphysis on the metaphysis. Three months after closed reduction and internal fixation with two cannulated screws, significant avascular necrosis had developed that resulted in loss of fixation and repeat slip. (*B*) AP view. (*C*) Lateral view. (*D*) Note the significant avascular necrosis at age 13 years, 11 months.

Table 1
Series of unstable SCFEs

Series	Loder et al [4]	Kallio et al [9]	Rattey et al [7]	Peterson et al [11]	Kennedy et al [10]	Phillips et al [19]	Gordon et al [17]	Tokmakova et al [12]
Year	1993	1995	1996	1997	2001	2001	2002	2003
Number of cases	30	34	26	91	27	14	16	36
AVN rate	14/30 (47%)	1/34 (3%)	4/26 (15%)	13/91 (14%)	4/27 (15%)	0/14 (0%)	2/16 (13%)	26/31 (84%)
Unintentional reduction occurred	Y	Y	N	—	Y	—	Y	—
Correlation with AVN		11 of 14			1 of 27			
Gender	N	—	—	↓ in girls	N	—	—	—
Race	N	—	—	Ø in African Americans	—	—	—	—
SCFE magnitude	N	—	↑ grade III	N	N	—	—	Y 13% (1/8)–I 70% (14/20)–II 75% (6/8)–III
Occurrence of reduction	N	N	N	N	N	—	Y	—
Magnitude of reduction	N	—	—	—	N	—	—	—
Time to reduction	Y <48 h (88% AVN (7 of 8) >48 h (32%) AVN (7 of 22)	—	—	≤24 h (7%) AVN (3 of 42) >24 h (20%) AVN (10 of 49)	N	Y <24 h (0% AVN, 0 of 14) >24 h (no patients)	Y <24 h (0% AVN, 0 of 10) >24 h (33% AVN, 2 of 6)	—
Number of pins	N	—	—	—	—	—	All used 2 screws	>AVN with multiple pins than 1 cannulated screw

risk for AVN [7,10]; in one series earlier reduction increased the risk for AVN [27]. Others believe that an early reduction is not detrimental and may actually be beneficial [11,17,19]. What about the magnitude of the SCFE? Does a more severe unstable SCFE have a higher risk for AVN? More severe SCFEs were noted to have an increased incidence of AVN in two series [7,12]; others noted no correlation between slip magnitude and AVN [10,11,27]. Does the number of fixation devices influence rotational stability and thus result in different rates of AVN? It seems intuitive that two screws give better rotational control of the unstable SCFE than one screw; however, the theoretic argument of improved rotational stability reducing vascular damage caused by rotation and the incidence of AVN has not been substantiated [7,27]. Tokmakova noted a higher prevalence of AVN with multiple pins compared with those fixed with a single central screw [12]. Another question is the effect of gender or race. Perthes disease, a childhood form of AVN of the proximal femur, is less common in girls and is extremely rare in African American children. Girls had a reduced incidence of AVN in one study [11]; gender differences were not noted by others [10,27]. AVN was less common in African American children in one study [11]; racial differences were not seen in another study [27]. What is not controversial in most investigators' minds is that the vascular damage and resultant AVN occurs at the moment of acute, abrupt slippage with obstruction or tearing of the superior and posterior retinacular vessels [4,8–12,17,18]. Because unstable SCFEs are uncommon, there are no large series in which these many different postulated risk factors can be analyzed rigorously from a statistic perspective. This requires further study [16]. It is hoped that a multicenter study recently started by Dr. Fred Dietz at the University of Iowa will answer this question. At present, the question of what is the best method of treatment for the unstable SCFE is unanswered.

In an effort to predict which children who have unstable SCFE will develop AVN, a pretreatment bone scan has been used by some. Rhoad and colleagues [8] noted that a pretreatment bone scan was an excellent predictor of AVN in the patient who has an unstable SCFE. In 10 of the children with unstable SCFEs in their series, 6 demonstrated ischemia by bone scan, and 5 of these 6 developed AVN. The real question, however, is what can the orthopaedic surgeon do to reduce the risk for AVN in the unstable SCFE? As noted, the literature is confusing and controversial. This has led to an increased renewal in emergent open reduction with femoral neck shortening after surgical dislocation. Ganz [28,29] has popularized surgical dislocation of the hip for different conditions. This approach involves a trochanteric osteotomy, surgical dislocation of the hip, preservation of the posterior vasculature, and shortening of the femoral neck with takedown of any interfering callus. This shortening and removal of callus theoretically reduces tension on the vascularity to the epiphysis; the epiphysis is then repositioned back on the metaphysis and is fixed with screw fixation. The goals are to reduce the rate of AVN and remove any metaphyseal impingement on the acetabulum. As yet, there are no published series in the English literature reporting the results of this approach with unstable SCFEs, although a few centers in this country are beginning to adapt this treatment in unstable SCFEs.

The role of osteotomy in the treatment of slipped capital femoral epiphysis

The role of osteotomy in the treatment of SCFE is controversial regarding indications, timing, and type of osteotomy. Some investigators believe that osteotomy should be strongly considered in all severe SCFEs [30–32], whereas others believe that osteotomy should be reserved only for functional issues [33,34]. Some believe that an osteotomy should be performed as the initial treatment in SCFE [30], whereas others believe that osteotomies should be considered only after physeal closure and assessment of the patient's function and hip rotation [33,35,36]. Finally, the location of the osteotomy is controversial; should it be at the level of the physis, more distal in the femoral neck, or in the intertrochanteric region?

Proximal femoral osteotomy initially makes the most orthopedic sense when selecting a treatment for a child who has SCFE. Although some series demonstrate low complication rates with osteotomy, most document a higher complication rate with osteotomy compared with in situ stabilization. These complications, primarily AVN (13% with cuneiform osteotomy) and chondrolysis (23% with intertrochanteric osteotomy, 16% with cuneiform osteotomy, 7% with basilar neck osteotomy), result in poor long-term outcomes. No long-term study has demonstrated an improved outcome in severe SCFEs treated with osteotomy compared with in situ fixation (primarily or after physeal closure) [5,37].

It is well known that the natural history of SCFE is gradual development of degenerative hip disease. In the long-term follow-up study of Carney and colleagues [5] at an average follow-up of 41 years, the risk for degenerative hip increased as the severity of the SCFE increased. The Iowa hip rating for the mild, moderate, and severe SCFEs was 89, 81, and 73 points, respectively. Similarly, children treated in situ did better than those who underwent realignment. The Iowa hip rating for the mild, moderate, and severe SCFEs was 77, 72, and 68 points when realigned, and 88, 88, and 85 points when not realigned. The realignment procedures used in those patients, however, were closed reductions in stable SCFEs, which we now know should not be performed, or osteotomies at a time when present-day improvements in intraoperative radiography and internal fixation did not exist. Does a realignment osteotomy performed today therefore have a better outcome than in the long-term study of Carney and colleagues, and if so, will an osteotomy using today's methods in a severe SCFE improve the natural history? This question is now being discussed among many pediatric orthopaedic surgeons, primarily because of increasing evidence of potential mechanical damage that can occur from the prominent femoral metaphysis in a severe SCFE on the acetabular cartilage [38–41].

In a series of 14 adolescent hips with SCFE, Leuning and colleagues [38] found that when the anterior femoral metaphysis was level with or extended past the epiphysis (Fig. 3), labral and acetabular cartilage damage occurred. The labral damage consisted of scars, tears, and erosions. The adjacent acetabular cartilage damage ranged from partial to full thickness loss. The femoral head cartilage was intact. These findings suggest that degenerative hip disease in children who have SCFE therefore can be triggered by early mechanical damage of the acetabular cartilage.

If a surgeon elects to reorient the epiphysis to normalize relations between the acetabulum and epiphysis, then multiple different osteotomy options are available. Proximal femoral osteotomy can be performed at several locations: (1) physeal (Fish or Dunn cuneiform osteotomy) [42,43], (2) basilar neck (eg, Abraham) [32,44], and (3) intertrochanteric/subtrochanteric level (Southwick, Imhäuser osteotomy) [33,45–47]. A physeal osteotomy at the level of deformity allows for maximum correction [42,43]. Its serious disadvantage is a high rate of AVN in most surgeons' hands. The few series with low AVN rates indicate that its success depends on the individual surgeon [42,43]. The Dunn procedure [42], which is essentially an open reduction of an SCFE, is popular in the United Kingdom and other countries with a British orthopedic influence. The basilar neck

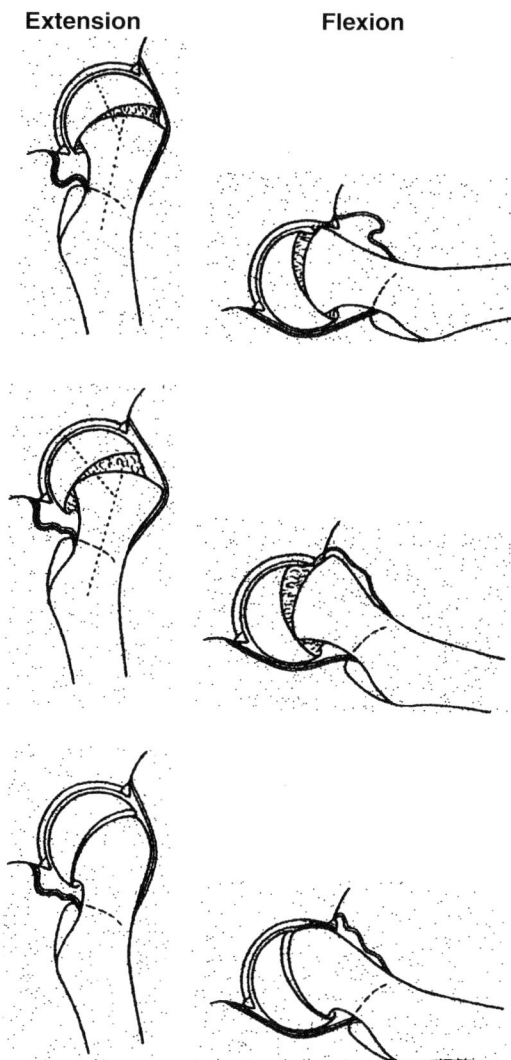

Fig. 3. Schematic lateral drawings of varying types of degrees of SCFE in extension and flexion. (*From* Leunig M, Casillas MM, Hamlet M, et al. Slipped capital femoral epiphysis. Early mechanical damage to the acetabular cartilage by a prominent femoral metaphysis. Acta Orthop Scand 2000;71(4):370–5; with permission.)

osteotomy has a lower risk for AVN, because it is done just distal to the entry site of the epiphyseal blood supply, yet close enough to the deformity for adequate correction [32,44]. Intertrochanteric/subtrochanteric osteotomies are compensatory and introduce a distal reverse deformity [45,48]. The advantage of this osteotomy is its low risk for AVN; however, it may not provide as much correction, can be complicated by chondrolysis, and fixation problems may occur. Later joint replacement arthroplasty is more difficult because of the distorted proximal femoral anatomy [49].

Recently the traditional Southwick type of osteotomy has been replaced by the simpler Imhäuser flexion intertrochanteric osteotomy [31,33,50] (Fig. 4). This osteotomy relies on the concept that the slip is essentially posterior [39,41,51] with secondary rotational deformity and minimal valgus or varus displacement. The results of such an osteotomy are disparate. Kartenbender and colleagues [33] reviewed 39 severe SCFEs treated with an Imhäuser osteotomy at an average follow-up of 23.4 years. Three patients had severe degenerative disease and two developed AVN. The number of excellent or good clinical results was 77%, whereas the excellent or good radiographic results using the Southwick classification were only 67%. The question becomes, will there be further deterioration after more time? By contrast, Parsch and colleagues [31] noted one AVN in 19 stable SCFEs >50°, yet concluded that they were unable to prove the advantage of osteotomy in late adult life. Schai and colleagues [30] reported on 51 patients at an average follow-up of 24 years who were treated by intertrochanteric osteotomy. At follow-up, 55% showed no radiographic or clinical signs of degenerative hip disease, 28% had moderate arthritis, and 17% had severe arthritis. They believed their results were superior to those treated by in situ fixation when they compared their results to those of Jerre [52]. Their results are at odds, however, with the long-term study of Carney and colleagues, in which realignment resulted in poorer results than those not realigned.

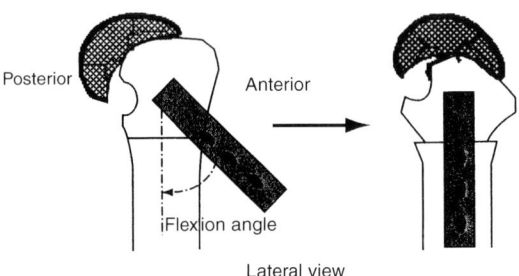

Fig. 4. The Imhäuser flexion closing wedge intertrochanteric osteotomy for a slipped capital femoral epiphysis. (*From* Kamegaya M, Saisu T, Ochiai N, et al. Preoperative assessment for intertrochanteric femoral osteotomies in severe chronic slipped capital femoral epiphysis using computed tomography. J Pediatr Orthop B 2005;14:71–8; with permission.)

Prophylactic fixation of the contralateral hip in children who have unilateral slipped capital femoral epiphysis

This is controversial in North America [53], although in Europe it is more commonly accepted [54]. In children who have underlying endocrine (eg, hypothyroidism) or metabolic (eg, renal failure) disorders, prophylactic fixation of the uninvolved hip should be strongly considered [53,55–58]. These types of SCFE, however, are infrequent compared with the idiopathic SCFE. In the idiopathic SCFE, the prevalence of bilaterality typically is quoted as 20% to 35% [59], with simultaneous presentation of bilaterality 10% to 20%. Hägglund quotes a prevalence of 61%, indicating that an additional 40% of patients who have SCFE at 16- to 66-year long-term follow-up demonstrate bilaterality [54]. Excluding the 61% prevalence figure, if all children who have unilateral SCFE underwent prophylactic fixation of the opposite hip, then 65% to 80% would have unnecessary surgery. This high rate of unnecessary surgery made it difficult to recommend prophylactic fixation.

In an attempt to answer this question, two investigators recently used decision analysis methods to answer this question. Different conclusions were reached, however, because of their methods of determining utility values. A utility value is the underlying concept in decision analysis; objective clinical outcome measures are assigned a utility value in the form of a linear scale. Schultz and colleagues [60] derived utility values from the literature for risks for chondrolysis, AVN (for those who underwent prophylactic fixation) and a sequential slip being detected during adolescence or later. They used these values in a model with two options: prophylactic fixation of the opposite hip or observation with close clinical and radiographic follow-up. They determined a threshold level for prophylactic fixation when considering the rates of sequential slip, rate of slip overlooked at follow-up, and complications associated with prophylactic fixation of the opposition (AVN and chondrolysis). The threshold rate for when the model favors observation is 18.1% for AVN and 21.6% for chondrolysis. Because the rates of AVN and chondrolysis are much less than 18.1% and 21.6%, they concluded that treatment of the contralateral hip with prophylactic fixation is beneficial for the long-term outcome of the uninvolved hip. Kocher and colleagues [61] reached the opposite conclusion. They used utility values obtained from questionnaires on patient preferences rather than complication rates, using a visual analog scale scored by 25 adolescent boys without SCFE. When determining utility values in this manner, the risks for prophylactic fixation outweigh potential benefits only when the probability of a contralateral SCFE is >27% or when reliable follow-up is not feasible. The decision to perform prophylactic fixation therefore depends on the probabilities of the various outcomes and on personal preferences. They advocate a patient–physician shared decision-making model in which outcome probabilities and patient preferences are considered to answer the question of prophylactic fixation. The real dilemma is how to determine when the risk for a contralateral SCFE in the idiopathic situation is >27%. This requires detailed knowledge regarding demographic predictors of bilaterality. Stasikelis and colleagues [62] studied the demographics and skeletal maturity of children who had unilateral SCFE to predict the development of bilateral involvement using a modified Oxford bone age score. They found that a score of 16 was associated with an 85% risk for contralateral involvement and a score of 21 with an 11% risk. Barrios and colleagues recently noted that the risk for bilaterality increased when the posterior slope angle of the capital femoral epiphysis was higher [63]. Further investigation into skeletal maturity and proximal femoral anatomic geometry should improve our knowledge regarding the risk for subsequent SCFE.

Fixation in the very young child with slipped capital femoral epiphysis

Most investigators today recommend single screw fixation for the typical adolescent with an SCFE. Segal and colleagues, however, documented growth disturbances of the proximal femur after this treatment in young children [64]. These disturbances are primarily coxa vara and coxa breva caused by premature proximal physeal arrest, with limitation of any epiphyseal and metaphyseal remodeling. In an effort to allow continued growth of the proximal femoral physis, several techniques have been used. One technique is simply using smooth Steinmann pins, allowing the epiphysis to grow off the pins, and then perform repeat fixation with longer pins [65–67]. Another method is the use of a hook pin [68] or modified screws. One modified screw technique [69] uses a cannulated screw with three threads rather than six. This allows for all the threads to be placed entirely in the epiphysis with a smooth shank crossing the physis. In one series of 10 SCFEs no screw loosening or growing off of the epiphysis was noted, yet remodeling and continued growth of the proximal femur occurred [69]. Another modification involves taking a fully threaded screw, removing the threads from the screw that will cross the physis, leaving threads that will engage the metaphysis, and then placing this modified screw across the physis in standard fashion [70]. There is no single correct solution to these rare and challenging cases of SCFE.

References

[1] Aadalen RJ, Weiner DS, Hoyt W, et al. Acute slipped capital femoral epiphysis. J Bone Joint Surg [Am] 1974;56A(7):1473–87.

[2] Fahey JJ, O'Brien ET. Acute slipped capital femoral epiphysis. J Bone Joint Surg [Am] 1965;47A(6):1105–27.

[3] Kallio PE, Paterson DC, Foster BK, et al. Classification in slipped capital femoral epiphysis. Sonographic assessment of stability and remodeling. Clin Orthop 1993;294:196–203.

[4] Loder RT, Richards BS, Shapiro PS, et al. Acute slipped capital femoral epiphysis: the importance of physeal stability. J Bone Joint Surg [Am] 1993;75A(8):1134–40.

[5] Carney BT, Weinstein SW, Noble J. Long-term follow-up of slipped capital femoral epiphysis. J Bone Joint Surg [Am] 1991;73A(5):667–74.

[6] Krahn TH, Canale ST, Beaty JH, et al. Long-term follow-up of patients with avascular necrosis after treatment of slipped capital femoral epiphysis. J Pediatr Orthop 1993;13:154–8.

[7] Rattey T, Piehl F, Wright JG. Acute slipped capital femoral epiphysis. Review of outcomes and rates of avascular necrosis. J Bone Joint Surg [Am] 1996;78A(3):398–402.

[8] Rhoad RC, Davidson RS, Heyman S, et al. Pretreatment bone scan in SCFE: a predictor of ischemia and avascular necrosis. J Pediatr Orthop 1999;19(2):164–8.

[9] Kallio PE, Mah ET, Foster BK, et al. Slipped capital femoral epiphysis. Incidence and assessment of physeal instability. J Bone Joint Surg [Br] 1995;77B(5):752–5.

[10] Kennedy JG, Hresko MT, Kasser JR, et al. Osteonecrosis of the femoral head associated with slipped capital femoral epiphysis. J Pediatr Orthop 2001;21(2):189–93.

[11] Peterson MD, Weiner DS, Green NE, et al. Acute slipped capital femoral epiphysis: the value and safety of urgent manipulative reduction. J Pediatr Orthop 1997;17:648–54.

[12] Tokmakova KP, Stanton RP, Mason DE. Factors influencing the development of osteonecrosis in patients treated for slipped capital femoral epiphysis. J Bone Joint Surg [Am] 2003;85A(5):798–801.

[13] Dietz FR. Traction reduction of acute and acute-on-chronic slipped capital femoral epiphysis. Clin Orthop 1994;302:101–10.

[14] Ballard J, Cosgrove AP. Anterior physeal separation. A sign indicating a high risk for avascular necrosis after slipped capital femoral epiphysis. J Bone Joint Surg [Br] 2002;84B(8):1176–9.

[15] Uglow MG, Clarke NMP. The management of slipped capital femoral epiphysis. J Bone Joint Surg [Br] 2004;86B(5):631–5.

[16] Mooney III JF, Sanders JO, Browne RH, et al. Management of unstable/acute slipped capital femoral epiphysis. Results of a survey of the POSNA membership. J Pediatr Orthop 2005;25(2):162–6.

[17] Gordon JE, Abrahams MS, Dobbs MB, et al. Early reduction, arthrotomy, and cannulated screw fixation in unstable slipped capital femoral epiphysis treatment. J Pediatr Orthop 2002;22(3):352–8.

[18] Maeda S, Kita A, Funayama K, et al. Vascular supply to slipped capital femoral epiphysis. J Pediatr Orthop 2001;21:664–7.

[19] Phillips SA, Griffiths WEG, Clarke NMP. The timing and reduction and stabilisation of the acute, unstable slipped upper femoral epiphysis. J Bone Joint Surg [Br] 2001;83B(7):1046–9.

[20] Sanders JO, Smith WJ, Stanley EA, et al. Progressive slippage after pinning for slipped capital femoral epiphysis. J Pediatr Orthop 2002;22:239–43.

[21] Karol LA, Doane RM, Cornicelli SF, et al. Single versus double screw fixation for treatment of slipped capital femoral epiphysis: a biomechanical analysis. J Pediatr Orthop 1992;12:741–5.

[22] Kibiloski LJ, Doane RM, Karol LA, et al. Biomechanical analysis of single- versus double-screw fixation in slipped capital femoral epiphysis at physiological load levels. J Pediatr Orthop 1994;14:627–30.

[23] Aronsson DD, Loder RT. Treatment of the unstable (acute) slipped capital femoral epiphysis. Clin Orthop 1996;322:99–110.

[24] Stanitski CL. Acute slipped capital femoral epiphysis: treatment alternatives. J Am Acad Orthop Surg 1994;2(2):96–106.

[25] Schmidt TL, Cimino WG, Seidel FG. Allograft epiphysiodesis for slipped capital femoral epiphysis. Clin Orthop 1996;322:61–76.

[26] Weiner DS, Weiner SD, Melby A. Anterolateral approach to the hip for bone graft epiphysiodesis in the treatment of slipped capital femoral epiphysis. J Pediatr Orthop 1988;8:349–52.

[27] Loder RT, Aronson DD, Greenfield ML. The epidemiology of bilateral slipped capital femoral epiphysis. A study of children in Michigan. J Bone Joint Surg [Am] 1993;75A(8):1141–7.

[28] Ganz R, Gill TJ, Gautier E, et al. Surgical dislocation of the adult hip. A technique with full access to the femoral head and acetabulum without the risk of avascular necrosis. J Bone Joint Surg [Br] 2001;83B(8):1119–24.

[29] Sienbenrock KA, Gautier E, Woo AKH, et al. Surgical dislocation of the femoral head for joint debridement and accurate reduction of fractures of the acetabulum. J Orthop Trauma 2002;16(8):543–52.

[30] Schai PA, Exner GU, Hansch O. Prevention of secondary coxarthrosis in slipped capital femoral epiphysis: a long-term follow-up study after corrective intertrochanteric osteotomy. J Pediatr Orthop B 1996;5:135–43.

[31] Parsch K, Bühl T, Weller S. Intertrochanteric corrective osteotomy for moderate and severe chronic slipped capital femoral epiphysis. J Pediatr Orthop B 1999;8(3):223–30.

[32] Abraham E, Garst J, Barmada R. Treatment of moderate to severe slipped capital femoral epiphysis with extracapsular base of neck osteotomy. J Pediatr Orthop 1993;13:294–302.

[33] Kartenbender K, Cordier W, Katthagen B-D. Long-term follow-up study after corrective Imhäuser osteotomy for severe slipped capital femoral epiphysis. J Pediatr Orthop 2000;20(6):749–56.

[34] Crawford AH. Role of osteotomy in the treatment of slipped capital femoral epiphysis. J Pediatr Orthop B 1996;5:102–9.

[35] DeRosa GP, Mullins RC, Kling Jr TF. Cuneiform osteotomy of the femoral neck in severe slipped capital femoral epiphysis. Clin Orthop 1996;322:48–60.

[36] Salvati EA, Robinson Jr HJ, O'Dowd TJ. Southwick osteotomy for severe chronic slipped capital femoral epiphysis: results and complications. J Bone Joint Surg [Am] 1980;62A(4):561–70.

[37] Ross PM, Lyne ED, Morawa LG. Slipped capital femoral epiphysis. Long term results after 10–38 years. Clin Orthop 1979;141:176–80.

[38] Leunig M, Casillas MM, Hamlet M, et al. Slipped capital femoral epiphysis. Early mechanical damage to the acetabular cartilage by a prominent femoral metaphysis. Acta Orthop Scand 2000;71(4):370–5.

[39] Rab GT. The geometry of slipped capital femoral epiphysis: implications for movement, impingement, and corrective osteotomy. J Pediatr Orthop 1999;19(4):419–24.

[40] Richolt JA, Teschner M, Everett PC, et al. Impingement simulation of the hip in SCFE using 3D models. Computer Aided Surg 1999;4(3):144–51.

[41] Cooperman DR, Charles LM, Pathria M, et al. Postmortem description of slipped capital femoral epiphysis. J Bone Joint Surg [Br] 1992;74B(4):595–9.

[42] Dunn DM, Angel JC. Replacement of the femoral head by open operation in severe adolescent slipping of the upper femoral epiphysis. J Bone Joint Surg [Br] 1978;60B(3):394–403.

[43] Fish JB. Cuneiform osteotomy of the femoral neck in the treatment of slipped capital femoral epiphysis. J Bone Joint Surg [Am] 1994;76A(1):46–59.

[44] Kramer WG, Craig WA, Noel S. Compensating osteotomy at the base of the femoral neck for slipped capital femoral epiphysis. J Bone Joint Surg [Am] 1976;58A(6):796–800.

[45] Southwick WO. Osteotomy through the lesser tro-

chanter for slipped capital femoral epiphysis. J Bone Joint Surg [Am] 1967;49A(5):807–35.
[46] Müller ME. Intertrochanteric osteotomy: indication, preoperative planning, technique. In: Schatzker J, editor. The intertrochanteric osteotomy. Berlin: Springer-Verlag; 1984. p. 25–66.
[47] Parsch K, Zehender H, Buhl T, et al. Intertrochanteric corrective osteotomy for moderate and severe chronic slipped capital femoral epiphysis. J Pediatr Orthop B 1999;8:223–30.
[48] Rao JP, Francis AM, Siwek CW. The treatment of chronic slipped capital femoral epiphysis by biplane osteotomy. J Bone Joint Surg [Am] 1984;66A(8): 1169–75.
[49] DeCoster TA, Incavo S, Frymoyer JW, et al. Hip arthroplasty after biplanar femoral osteotomy. J Arthroplasty 1989;4(1):79–86.
[50] Kamegaya M, Saisu T, Ochiai N, et al. Preoperative assessment for intertrochanteric femoral osteotomies in severe chronic slipped capital femoral epiphysis using computed tomography. J Pediatr Orthop B 2005; 14:71–8.
[51] Gelberman RH, Cohen MS, Shaw BA, et al. The association of femoral retroversion with slipped capital femoral epiphysis. J Bone Joint Surg [Am] 1986; 68A(7):1000–7.
[52] Jerre T. A study in slipped upper femoral epiphysis with special reference to late functional and roentgenological results and the value of closed reduction. Acta Orthop Scand 1950;6(Suppl).
[53] Castro Jr FP, Bennett JT, Doulens K. Epidemiological perspective on prophylactic pinning in patients with unilateral slipped capital femoral epiphysis. J Pediatr Orthop 2000;20(6):745–8.
[54] Hägglund G. The contralateral hip in slipped capital femoral epiphysis. J Pediatr Orthop B 1996;5:158–61.
[55] Loder RT, Wittenberg B, DeSilva G. Slipped capital femoral epiphysis associated with endocrine disorders. J Pediatr Orthop 1995;15:349–56.
[56] Loder RT, Hensinger RN. Slipped capital femoral epiphysis associated with renal failure osteodystrophy. J Pediatr Orthop 1997;17:205–11.
[57] Loder RT, Greenfield MLVH. Clinical characteristics of children with atypical and idiopathic slipped capital femoral epiphysis: description of the age-weight test and implications for further diagnostic investigation. J Pediatr Orthop 2001;21(4):481–7.

[58] Jerre R, Billing L, Hansson G, et al. The contralateral hip in patients primarily treated for unilateral slipped upper femoral epiphysis. J Bone Joint Surg [Br] 1994; 76B(4):563–7.
[59] Loder RT. Continents ACFOCA. The demographics of slipped capital femoral epiphysis. An international multicenter study. Clin Orthop 1996;322:8–27.
[60] Schultz WR, Weinstein JN, Weinstein SL, et al. Prophylactic pinning of the contralateral hip in slipped capital femoral epiphysis. Evaluation of long-term outcome for the contralateral hip with use of decision analysis. J Bone Joint Surg [Am] 2002;84A(8):1305–14.
[61] Kocher MS, Bishop JA, Hresko MT, et al. Prophylactic pinning of the contralateral hip after unilateral slipped capital femoral epiphysis. J Bone Joint Surg [Am] 2004;86A(12):2658–65.
[62] Stasikelis PJ, Sullivan CM, Phillips WA, et al. Slipped capital femoral epiphysis. Prediction of contralateral involvement. J Bone Joint Surg [Am] 1996;78A(8): 1149–55.
[63] Barrios C, Blasco MA, Blasco MC, et al. Posterior slipping angle of the capital femoral epiphysis. A predictor of bilaterality in slipped capital femoral epiphysis. J Pediatr Orthop 2005;25(4):445–9.
[64] Segal LS, Davidson RS, Robertson WWJ, et al. Growth disturbance after pinning of juvenile slipped capital femoral epiphysis. J Pediatr Orthop 1991;11: 631–7.
[65] Loder RT, Hensinger RN, Alburger PD, et al. Slipped capital femoral epiphysis associated with radiation therapy. J Pediatr Orthop 1998;18:630–6.
[66] Walker SJ, Whiteside LA, McAlister WH, et al. Slipped capital femoral epiphysis following radiation and chemotherapy. Clin Orthop 1981;159:186–93.
[67] Oppenheim WL, Bowen RE, McDonough PW, et al. Outcome of slipped capital femoral epiphysis in renal osteodystrophy. J Pediatr Orthop 2003;23: 169–74.
[68] Hansson LI. Osteosynthesis with the hook-pin in slipped capital femoral epiphysis. Acta Orthop Scand 1982;53:87–96.
[69] Guzzanti V, Falciglia F, Stanitski CL. Slipped capital femoral epiphysis in skeletally immature patients. J Bone Joint Surg [Br] 2004;85B(5):731–6.
[70] Hartjen CA, Koman LA. Treatment of slipped capital femoral epiphysis resulting from juvenile renal osteodystrophy. J Pediatr Orthop 1990;10:551–4.

Fractures of the Hip in Children

James H. Beaty, MD

Department of Orthopaedic Surgery, Campbell Clinics, University of Tennessee, 1211 Union Avenue, Suite 510, Memphis, TN 38104, USA

Fractures of the hip are rare injuries in children, accounting for fewer than 1% of all pediatric fractures [1–4]; most are caused by high-energy trauma, with only a few caused by minor trauma, trivial trauma, or pathologic conditions [2,5–9]. Perhaps because of their rarity, management principles remain largely unchanged from early reports. It is not the frequency of hip fracture in children, or controversies about new treatment methods, that make them important, but rather the frequency of potentially devastating complications that accompany them: osteonecrosis, coxa vara, premature physeal closure, limb-length discrepancy, and nonunion [2,4–6,10,11].

Anatomy

Many of the complications associated with hip fractures in children occur because of the unique anatomy of the hip in skeletally immature individuals. A single proximal physis present at birth transforms into two discrete physes (capital femoral and greater trochanteric), appearing at about 4 to 6 months and 4 years of age, respectively. These physes fuse around the age of 16 years in boys and 14 years in girls [12–14]. The persistent cartilaginous bridge and the tenuous blood supply to the posterosuperior aspect of the femoral neck make the proximal aspect of the femur highly vulnerable to physeal damage, growth arrest, and subsequent deformity after a fracture of the hip.

The vulnerability of the blood supply to the proximal femoral epiphysis has been thoroughly documented by Chung [15], Odgen [16], and Trueta [17] who found that the primary blood supply to the femoral head from birth until the age of about 4 years is from the medial and lateral circumflex arteries that traverse the femoral neck (Fig. 1). Then the metaphyseal blood supply becomes negligible and the two (posterosuperior and posteroinferior) retinacular systems of the medial femoral circumflex artery become the primary blood supply to the epiphysis. After the age of 8 or 9 years, the vessels of the ligamentum teres make a more important contribution to the blood supply of the femoral head and, at puberty, the anastomosis between the epiphyseal, metaphyseal, and ligamentum blood supplies is re-established [17]. The femoral head is most susceptible to vascular compromise because the multiple channels of blood supply in an immature individual change with age to a limited blood supply in a mature individual.

Ogden [16] noted that, because the branches of the medial circumflex artery traverse the capsule at the level of the insertion into the intertrochanteric notch, capsulotomy does not affect the blood supply to the femoral head if the capsular incision does not extend to the intertrochanteric notch. This finding supports the clinical observation that the risk of osteonecrosis is directly affected by the degree of initial trauma and displacement and the age of the patient rather than by the type of treatment [2,5,8,9,18–20].

Mechanism of injury

Most (85%–90%) hip fractures in children and adolescents are caused by severe high-energy trauma, and approximately 30% are associated with other major injuries [21–24]. Intra-abdominal or intrapelvic

E-mail address: jbeaty@campbellclinic.com

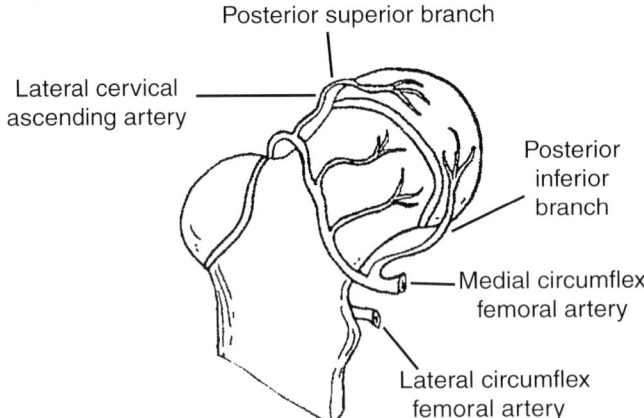

Fig. 1. Arterial supply of the proximal femur. Capital femoral epiphysis and physis are supplied by the medial circumflex artery through two retinacular vessel systems: posterosuperior and posteroinferior. The lateral circumflex artery supplied the greater trochanter and the lateral portion of the proximal femoral physis and a small area of the anteromedial metaphysis. (*From* Blaiser RD, Hughes LO. Fractures and traumatic dislocations of the hip in children. In: Beaty JH, Kasser JR, editors. Rockwood and Wilkins' fractures in children. 5th edition. Philadelphia: JB Lippincott; 2001. p. 917; with permission.)

visceral injuries and head injuries are the most common associated injuries; hip dislocations, pelvic fractures, and femoral shaft fractures occur less frequently. Hip fractures in infants may be associated with child abuse; they often are associated with a pathologic condition, such as unicameral bone cyst, aneurysmal bone cyst, osteogenesis imperfecta, fibrous dysplasia, myelomeningocele, or osteopenia [25–27].

Diagnosis

Most hip fractures are easily diagnosed. The patient reports severe pain and a history of high-energy trauma and usually is unable actively to move the limb; even passive motion may be limited by pain. With a displaced fracture, the patient holds the injured limb laterally rotated and slightly adducted and the limb appears shortened. If the femoral head is dislocated, the limb is held in flexion, adduction, and internal rotation. Nondisplaced fractures may not produce such obvious signs, and only mild discomfort may be caused by passive range of motion of the extremity. The patient may even be able to walk with little pain. Because of the lack of marked signs or symptoms, nondisplaced fractures or stress fractures may not be diagnosed at initial evaluation.

Anteroposterior and lateral radiographs provide information about the type of fracture (classification); direction of the fracture line; amount of displacement; degree of varus; and location of the femoral epiphysis. MRI is useful for the diagnosis of nondisplaced or stress fractures and also may supply additional information about femoral head viability [28,29]; however, treatment should not be delayed to obtain MRI scans.

Classification

The most widely used classification of hip fractures in children is that of Delbet [30,31] (Fig. 2), in which four types are described based on location: type I, transepiphyseal, with or without femoral head dislocation; type II, transcervical, displaced or nondisplaced; type III, cervicotrochanteric, displaced or nondisplaced; and type IV, intertrochanteric. This classification has been proved to be helpful in determining treatment and predicting complications and outcomes.

Type I fractures

Type I fractures (transepiphyseal separations) are the least common type of hip fractures in children (<10%); they occur more often in young children than do the other three types [1–9]. This injury occurs predominantly in two age groups: infants and young children (younger than 2 years) and children aged 5 to 10 years. In young children, severe trauma is required to produce this type of fracture; in neonates, this injury is known as "proximal femoral epiphysiolysis" and can be caused by a difficult delivery or by child abuse

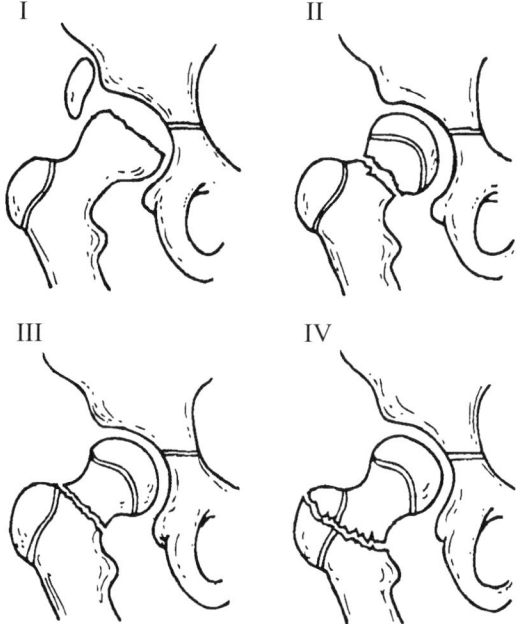

Fig. 2. Delbet classification of fractures of the head and neck of the femur in children. Type I: transepiphyseal separation, with or without dislocation of the femoral head. Type II: nondisplaced or displaced transcervical fracture. Type III: nondisplaced or displaced cervicotrochanteric fracture. Type IV: intertrochanteric fracture. (*From* Hughes LO, Beaty JH. Current concepts review: fractures of the head and neck of the femur in children. J Bone Joint Surg Am 1994;76:284; with permission.)

in an infant. This fracture has been reported to occur during attempted closed reduction of a traumatic hip dislocation with a nondisplaced physeal fracture in adolescents [32–34].

Diagnosis may be difficult in a newborn in which the femoral head is not ossified. This injury should be suspected in an infant who holds the extremity flexed, abducted, and externally rotated; the extremity may be short and without any spontaneous movement. If plain radiographs are unrevealing, ultrasonography can aid in the diagnosis. In children and adolescents, the diagnosis is based on a history of severe trauma, physical examination, and radiographs.

Dislocation of the femoral head occurs with approximately 50% of type I fractures (Fig. 3), making this type the most commonly associated with osteonecrosis and premature physeal closure (up to 100% of those with type I fractures with dislocation) [2,21,23,35]. Associated injuries, most often pelvic fractures, also are common in patients with type I hip fractures.

Patients younger than 2 to 3 years at the time of injury have a better prognosis than older children, possibly because the remodeling potential is better in younger patients.

Type II fractures

Type II (transcervical) fractures are the most common hip fractures in children and adolescents (40%–50%) [1–9]. Most are caused by severe trauma, such as a fall from a height, motor-vehicle accident, or pedestrian-vehicle accident, and over half

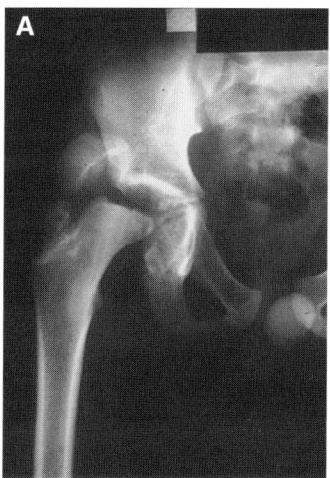
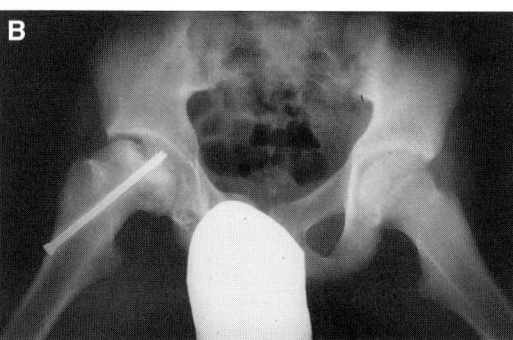

Fig. 3. (*A*) Type I fracture with dislocation of the femoral head. (*B*) Two years after fixation, osteonecrosis of the femoral head is apparent.

are displaced. Three peak ages have been identified for type II fractures: 2 to 4 years of age, 8 and 9 years of age, and 12 and 13 years of age [36].

The reported prevalences of osteonecrosis after type II fractures range from 16% to 78% [2,5,7,9,19–21,35]. Results of nondisplaced type II fractures are better, regardless of treatment method, than are results of displaced fractures, with which osteonecrosis is much more frequent. The likelihood of osteonecrosis has been linked to the initial displacement of the fracture fragments, but osteonecrosis does occur after nondisplaced fractures [2,5,8,18,37].

Type III fractures

Type III (cervicotrochanteric) fractures are the second most common type of hip fractures in children (25%–30%) [1–9]. Severe trauma is required to produce this injury in a child. Osteonecrosis (25%), premature physeal closure (25%), and coxa vara (14%) are frequent after displaced type III fractures; complications are uncommon after nondisplaced fractures.

Type IV fractures

Type IV (intertrochanteric) fractures account for 6% to 15% of hip fractures in children [1–9]. Osteonecrosis is infrequent after these fractures (<10%), and these fractures have the best overall outcomes.

Treatment

Type I

For type I fracture without dislocation, gentle closed reduction is followed by fixation with smooth pins (children <4 years old) or cannulated screws (older children and adolescents) (see Fig. 3). In children younger than 2 years of age, closed reduction and application of a hip-spica cast without internal fixation may be adequate if the reduction seems stable [38].

Closed reduction of a type I fracture with dislocation of the femoral head from the acetabulum usually is not possible; a single, gentle attempt may be made, but multiple attempts should be avoided. Open reduction and pin and screw fixation are indicated if closed reduction is unsuccessful. Some authors have recommended immediate open reduction of transepiphyseal fractures with femoral head dislocation to preserve any remaining capsular attachments and intact blood supply [39,40]. The operative approach is determined by the direction of the dislocation: anterior approach for an anterior dislocation, posterior approach for a posterior dislocation. CT scanning is helpful for verification of the dislocation and determination of its direction.

Type II fractures

To minimize the risk of late complications (malunion, delayed union, nonunion, coxa vara), type II fractures should be treated with anatomic reduction and stable fixation. Internal fixation of both nondisplaced and displaced, with avoidance of penetration of the physis with the pin if possible, is recommended by most authors [2,8,21,24]. Cannulated screws should be inserted short of the physis if possible; however, this is not always possible, and the emphasis should be on obtaining stable fixation of the fracture even if physeal penetration is necessary (Fig. 4). Later treatment of a leg-length discrepancy is preferable to a malunion or nonunion that occurs because of inadequate fixation. Gentle closed reduc-

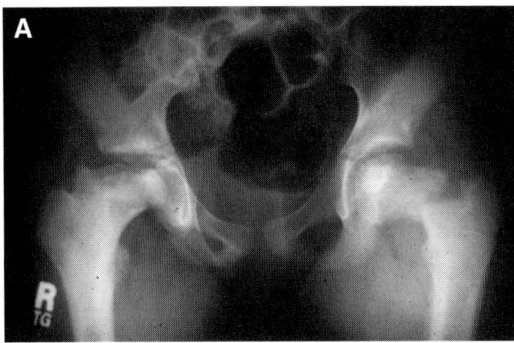
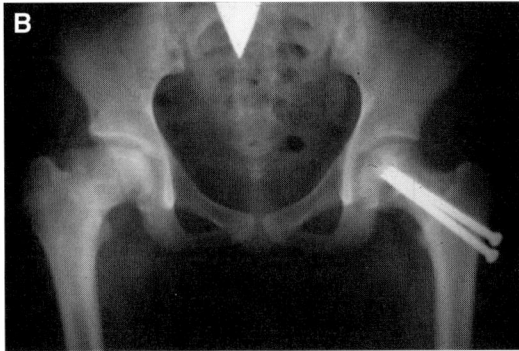

Fig. 4. (*A*) Type II fracture in a patient with Gaucher's disease. (*B*) Six months after fixation with 6.5-mm cannulated screws.

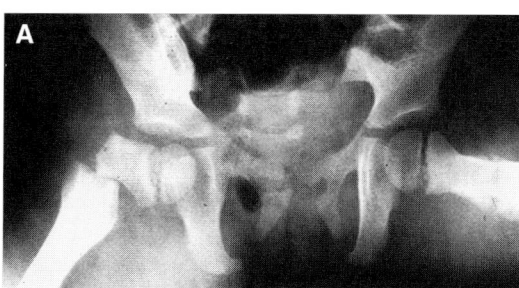
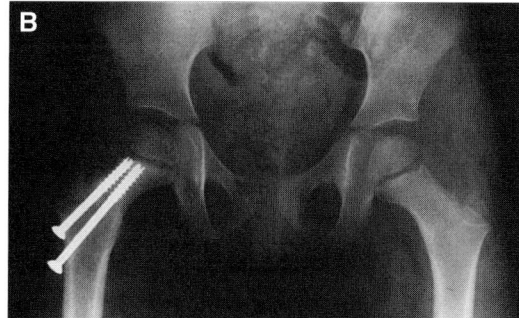

Fig. 5. (*A*) Type III fracture in a 5-year-old girl. (*B*) One year after fixation with 4-mm cannulated screws.

tion of displaced fractures can be attempted with longitudinal traction, abduction, and internal rotation, but this often is unsuccessful and open reduction frequently is required for type II fractures. Spica-cast treatment has been suggested for nondisplaced type II fractures [19,35,41], but close follow-up is necessary to detect loss of reduction if this method is used; I generally prefer hip aspiration and percutaneous screw fixation for nondisplaced type II fractures and open reduction and internal fixation for markedly displaced fractures.

Type III fractures

Nondisplaced type III fractures in young children (younger than 6 years old) can be treated with an abduction spica cast after a period of traction, but close follow-up is mandatory to detect fracture displacement. Nondisplaced fractures in older children and adolescents and all displaced type III fractures require internal fixation with cannulated screws (Fig. 5) or a hip-screw and side-plate construct.

Type IV fractures

Good results have been reported after closed reduction, traction, and spica cast immobilization of both undisplaced and displaced intertrochanteric fractures. Inadequate reduction, however, can lead to a varus malunion. Older children (more than 8 years of age), especially those with multiple injuries, should be treated with open reduction and internal fixation, avoiding the physis if possible (Fig. 6).

General treatment considerations

No matter which type of fracture is involved, when operative treatment is indicated, several other factors must be considered. Perhaps the most im-

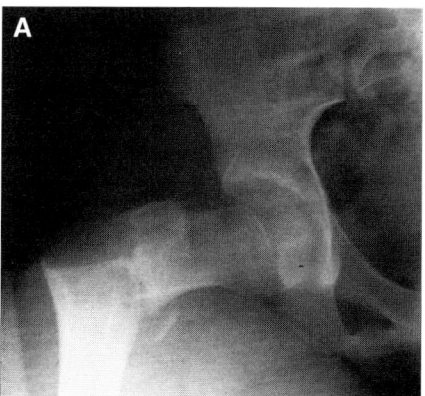
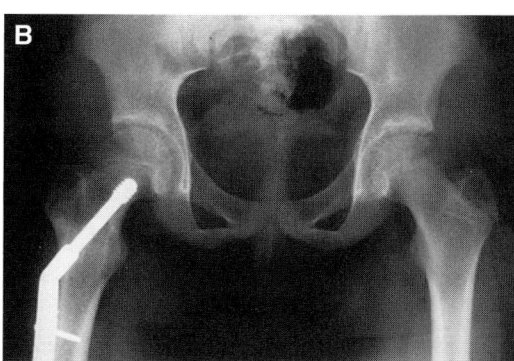

Fig. 6. (*A*) Type IV fracture in a 12-year-old child. (*B*) One year after open reduction and internal fixation with an intermediate hip compression screw. (*From* Hughes LO, Beaty JH. Current concepts review: fractures of the head and neck of the femur in children. J Bone Joint Surg Am 1994;76:288; with permission.)

portant consideration is age of the patient. For younger and smaller patients, a radiolucent operating table should be used rather than a fracture table, which is more appropriate for older and larger children and adolescents. For internal fixation of types I, II, or III fractures, smooth pins can be used in infants; cannulated 4-mm screws in children younger than 8 years; and 6.5-mm screws (Smith-Nephew, Memphis, TN) in adolescents. Pediatric-size hip compression screws are used for fixation of type IV fractures in children; adult-size devices can be used in adolescents. Predrilling and pretapping are necessary for screw insertion because of the dense, hard bone of the femoral neck in children.

A hip spica cast may be used to supplement internal fixation in all children younger than 10 years; no postoperative cast is needed for adolescents 12 years or older. In patients between the ages of 10 and 12 years, the need for a postoperative hip spica cast is based on the stability of the fracture fixation and the expected compliance of the patient; if either is questionable, a cast should be used for a brief period of time.

Rigid, stable fixation of the fracture is more important than preservation of the physis. If stability is questionable, the internal fixation device should extend into the femoral head for rigid, stable fixation regardless of the fracture type or age of the child. The contribution of the proximal femoral physis to the length of the extremity is only 13% (3–4 mm a year), and premature physeal closure alone generally does not result in marked deformity or limb-length discrepancy. When premature physeal closure occurs with osteonecrosis, however, especially in a young child, severe discrepancies can develop.

Complications

Osteonecrosis

The most common and most devastating complication of hip fractures in children is osteonecrosis of the femoral head (Fig. 7), with an overall prevalence of 17% to 47%. The observation of Ingram and Bachynski [5] in 1953 that the occurrence of osteonecrosis is directly related to the amount of initial fracture displacement and to the compromise of the blood supply at the time of fracture is still valid. Numerous reports have confirmed that osteonecrosis occurs much more often after displaced fractures (90%) than after nondisplaced fractures, and the type of fracture treatment has not been proved to have an effect on the development of osteonecrosis. Immedi-

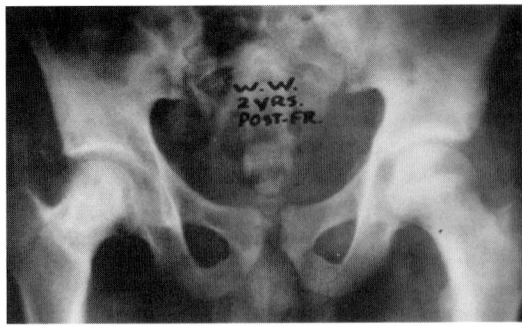

Fig. 7. Type 2 osteonecrosis of the femoral head 24 months after type I fracture. (*From* Canale ST, Beaty JH. Pelvic and hip fractures. In: Rockwood Jr CA, Wilkins KE, Beaty JH, editors. Fractures in children. 4th edition. Philadelphia: Lippincott Raven; 1996. p. 1170; with permission.)

ate open reduction and internal fixation with evacuation of the intracapsular hematoma has been recommended to decrease the risk of osteonecrosis, but the effectiveness of this remains unclear. Several authors have reported that decompressive hip arthrotomy reduces the risk of osteonecrosis [42–45], but Gerber and coworkers [46], in a review of hip fractures in children at seven Swiss hospitals, were unable to demonstrate an improvement in the occurrence of osteonecrosis, and Pape and coworkers [23] reported 89% good or fair results without capsulotomy in their 28 patients. Because hip decompression is relatively easy to perform and is associated with minimal complications, and may indeed lower the risk of osteonecrosis, it should be considered after reduction and fixation to minimize the accumulation of fracture hematoma. The hip joint can be aspirated with an 18-gauge needle through a subadductor approach at the time of reduction and fixation or a small capsulotomy can be made along the anterior femoral neck.

Although early reduction (within 24 hours) has been shown to improve outcomes in adults with hip fractures, few studies have directly compared early and late treatment in children [11,42]. Pförringer and Rosemeyer [20] reported better outcomes in children and adolescents with early operative treatment (within 36 hours) than in those treated later. Other factors associated with an increased risk of osteonecrosis are a type I or II fracture and an age of 10 years or more at the time of injury.

Pain and limitation of motion because of synovitis may be the first signs of osteonecrosis. Radiographic evidence may be apparent as early as 6 to 8 weeks after fracture, including lack of development or osteoporosis of the femoral head and widening of the cartilage space followed by fragmentation and gross deformity of the femoral head. Bone scanning at 3 to 4 months after fracture and again at 12 months after fracture has been recommended to detect osteonecrosis, which usually develops within the first year after the injury [2]. MRI is the most sensitive test to confirm the diagnosis and also defines the extent of femoral head and neck involvement, but may not be useful if stainless steel internal fixation has been used.

Ratliff [9] described three types of femoral head osteonecrosis: type I, total osteonecrosis of the entire femoral capital epiphysis and proximal neck; type II, metaphyseal osteonecrosis from the level of the fracture to the physis; and type III, partial femoral head osteonecrosis. Type I, the most severe, also is the most common and results from disruption of the lateral epiphyseal and metaphyseal vessels. Other classifications of femoral head osteonecrosis include those developed by Ficat and Arlet [47]; Marcus and coworkers [48]; Steinberg and coworkers [49]; Plakseychuk and coworkers [50] (Pittsburgh classification); and the Association Research Circulation Osseous [51]. The use of multiple classification systems makes comparison of studies difficult, and no system has been proved to be superior in aiding treatment decision-making or prognosis, and the Ratliff system continues to be used by most pediatric orthopedists.

Approximately 60% of patients who develop femoral head osteonecrosis have poor results, with pain, limited range of motion, and deformities of the femoral head and proximal femur [1,2,8,21,35]. No treatment method has been proved to treat femoral head osteonecrosis successfully in children. Recommended treatments include observation; bed rest; non–weight-bearing [52,53]; and operative procedures, such as soft tissue releases about the hip for flexion and adduction contractures, core decompression [54,55], vascularized fibular grafting [56,57], hemiarthroplasty [58,59], arthroplasty, and arthrodesis [60]. Dean and coworkers [56] reported promising results in 50 pediatric patients after free vascularized fibular grafting, noting a lower rate of conversion to total hip arthroplasty in pediatric patients (16%) than in adult patients (25%). They also noted that the radiographic appearance of the femoral head in children and adolescents had less correlation with their clinical symptoms than in adults.

Coxa vara

Coxa vara occurs after 10% to 30% hip fractures and may be the result of malreduction (varus) of the fracture, loss of reduction, delayed union or nonunion, osteonecrosis, or premature closure of the proximal femoral physis with overgrowth of the greater trochanter [1,2,8,21,35]. It is more frequent and more severe after closed reduction and cast immobilization than after closed reduction and internal fixation. Severe coxa vara shortens the affected extremity, causes an abductor or gluteal lurch, and may result in late degenerative changes about the hip. Progressive remodeling of coxa vara deformity can be expected in very young children and those in whom the neck-shaft angle is 110 degrees or more. Subtrochanteric valgus osteotomy should be considered for children older than 8 years of age and for those with neck-shaft angles of less than 110 degrees (Fig. 8).

Premature physeal closure

Premature physeal closure has been reported after 5% to 65% of hip fractures in children [1,2,8,21,35]. The frequency increases when internal fixation crosses the physis or when osteonecrosis is present. Because the capital femoral physis contributes only 13% of the growth of the entire extremity and normally closes earlier than most of the other physes in the lower extremity, shortening is usually less than 2 cm except in very young children. Children with premature physeal closure should be followed with sequential limb-length scanograms and wrist radiographs to determine bone age; if the limb-length discrepancy is projected to be 2.5 cm or more, contralateral epiphysiodesis can be done.

Nonunion

Nonunion is infrequent after hip fractures in children, occurring in 6% to 10%, and is related to

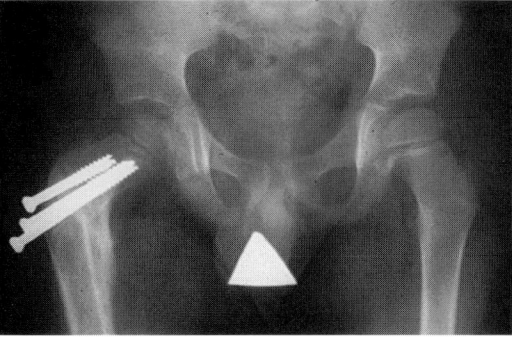

Fig. 8. Coxa vara deformity in a 5-year-old after a type III fracture. Subtrochanteric osteotomy was later required. (*From* Canale ST, Beaty JH. Pelvic and hip fractures. In: Rockwood Jr CA, Wilkins KE, Beaty JH, editors. Fractures in children. 4th edition. Philadelphia: Lippincott Raven; 1996. p. 1173; with permission.)

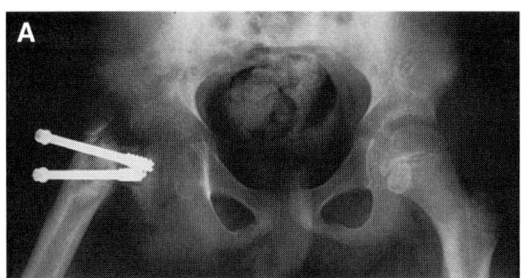 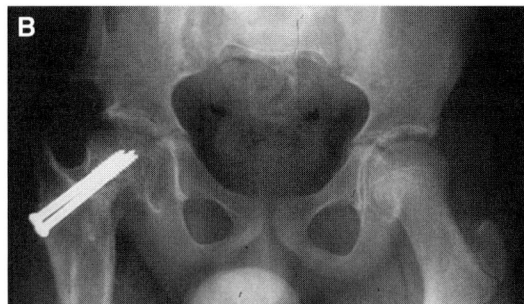

Fig. 9. (*A*) Nonunion of a type III fracture 3 months after cannulated screw fixation. (*B*) Union obtained after subtrochanteric osteotomy, bone grafting, and screw fixation; mild osteonecrosis is present. (*From* Canale ST, Beaty JH. Pelvic and hip fractures. In: Rockwood Jr CA, Wilkins KE, Beaty JH, editors. Fractures in children. 4th edition. Philadelphia: Lippincott Raven; 1996. p. 1175; with permission.)

the attainment and maintenance of an adequate anatomic reduction [1,2,8,21,35]. Rates of nonunion of hip fractures in children have been greatly reduced by the more frequent use of internal fixation. Unlike osteonecrosis and coxa vara, for which a period of observation is appropriate, nonunion should be treated operatively as soon as possible. Subtrochanteric valgus osteotomy can be done to make the nonunion more horizontal and to allow compressive vertical forces to aid in union. Bone grafts can be used if necessary to augment the osteotomy, and internal fixation should be used across the nonunion site; a spica cast is worn for 12 weeks after osteotomy (Fig. 9).

Other complications

Infection is relatively rare after hip fractures in children and adolescents, generally reported to occur in 1% to 10% of patients and most often after open reductions. Taylor and McHale [61] reported a deep infection after percutaneous pin fixation of a femoral neck fracture in a 12 year old.

Chondrolysis after hip fractures was reported in seven patients by Forlin and coworkers [62], but has not been reported by other investigators. This may have represented degenerative joint disease from persistent pin penetration in some patients. Late separation of a physis after fixation of a femoral neck fracture also has been reported [63].

Summary

Fractures of the hip are uncommon in children, and their importance is related not to the frequency of the injury but to the frequency of complications. Many of these complications can be minimized or avoided by anatomic reduction and internal fixation. Open reduction frequently is necessary to obtain a stable, anatomic reduction. Regardless of the age of the child, stable fixation of the fracture must be given priority over preservation of the proximal femoral physis. The development of osteonecrosis, however, is most likely related to the severity of the initial injury and is largely unaffected by treatment of the fracture.

References

[1] Azouz EM, Karamitsos C, Reed MH, et al. Types and complications of femoral neck fractures in children. Pediatr Radiol 1993;23:415–20.

[2] Hughes LO, Beaty JH. Current concepts review: fractures of the head and neck of the femur in children. J Bone Joint Surg Am 1994;76:283–92.

[3] Morrisy RT. Fractured hip in childhood. Instr Course Lect 1984;33:229–41.

[4] Quick TJ, Eastwood DM. Pediatric fractures and dislocations of the hip and pelvis. Clin Orthop 2005; 432:87–96.

[5] Ingram AJ, Bachynski B. Fractures of the hip in children: treatment and results. J Bone Joint Surg Am 1953;35:867–87.

[6] Kay SP, Hall JE. Fracture of the femoral neck in children and its complications. Clin Orthop 1971;80: 53–71.

[7] Lam SF. Fractures of the neck of the femur in children. J Bone Joint Surg Am 1971;53:1165–79.

[8] Morsy HA. Complications of fracture of the neck of the femur in children: a long-term follow-up study. Injury 2001;32:45–51.

[9] Ratliff SHC. Fractures of the neck of the femur in children. J Bone Joint Surg Br 1962;44:528–42.

[10] Bagatur AE, Zorer G. Complications associated with surgically treated hip fractures in children. J Pediatr Orthop 2002;11B:218–28.

[11] Flynn JM, Wong KL, Yeg GL, et al. Displaced fractures of the hip in children: management by early operation and immobilisation in a hip spica cast. J Bone Joint Surg Br 2002;84:108–12.

[12] Canale ST, King RE. Pelvic and hip fractures. Part II. Fractures of the hip. In: Rockwood Jr CA, Wilkins KE, King RE, editors. Fracture in children. 3rd edition. Philadelphia: JB Lippincott; 1991. p. 1046–120.

[13] Herring JA, McCarthy RE. Instructional case: fracture dislocation of the capital femoral epiphysis. J Pediatr Orthop 1986;6:112–4.

[14] Ogden JA. Hip development and vascularity: relationship to chondro-osseous trauma in the growing child. In: Salvati EA, editor. The hip: proceedings of the Ninth Open Scientific Meeting of the Hip Society. St. Louis: CV Mosby; 1981. p. 139–87.

[15] Chung SMK. The arterial supply of the developing proximal end of the human femur. J Bone Joint Surg Am 1976;58:961–70.

[16] Ogden JA. Changing patterns of proximal femoral vascularity. J Bone Joint Surg Am 1974;56:941–50.

[17] Trueta J. The normal vascular anatomy of the human femoral head during growth. J Bone Joint Surg Br 1957;39:358–94.

[18] Canale ST. Fractures of the hip in children and adolescents. Orthop Clin North Am 1990;21:341–52.

[19] Heiser JM, Oppenheim WL. Fracture of the hip in children: a review of forty cases. Clin Orthop 1980;149:177–84.

[20] Pförringer W, Rosemeyer B. Fractures of the hip in children and adolescents. Acta Orthop Scand 1980;51:91–108.

[21] Canale ST, Bourland WK. Fracture of the neck and intertrochanteric region of the femur in children. J Bone Joint Surg Am 1977;59:431–43.

[22] Mirdad T. Fractures of the neck of the femur in children: an experience at the Aseer Central Hospital, Abba, Saudi Arabia. Injury 2002;33:823–7.

[23] Pape HC, Krettek C, Friedrich A, et al. Long-term outcome in children with fractures of the proximal femur after high-energy trauma. J Trauma 1999;46:58–64.

[24] Swiontkowski MF, Winquist RA. Displaced hip fractures in children and adolescents. J Trauma 1986;26:384–8.

[25] Ahn JL, Park JS. Pathological fractures secondary to unicameral bone cysts. Int Orthop 1994;18:20–2.

[26] Morrissy RT. Hip fractures in children. Clin Orthop 1980;152:202–10.

[27] Quinlan WR, Brady PG, Regan BF. Fracture of the neck of the femur in childhood. Injury 1980;11:242–7.

[28] Ingari JV, Smith DK, Aufdemorte TB, et al. Anatomic significance of magnetic resonance imaging findings in hip fracture. Clin Orthop 1996;332:209–14.

[29] Speer KP, Spritzer CE, Harrelson JM, et al. Magnetic resonance imaging of the femoral head after acute intracapsular fracture of the femoral neck. J Bone Joint Surg Am 1990;72:98–103.

[30] Colonna PC. Fractures off the neck of the femur in children. Am J Surg 1928;6:793–7.

[31] Delbet MP. Fractures due col de femur. Bull Mem Soc Chir 1908;35:387–9.

[32] Blaiser RD, Hughes LO. Fractures and traumatic dislocations of the hip in children. In: Beaty JH, Kasser JR, editors. Rockwood and Wilkins' fractures in children. 5th edition. Philadelphia: JB Lippincott; 2001. p. 913–40.

[33] Gaudinez RF, Heinrich SD. Transphyseal fracture of the capital femoral epiphysis. Orthopedics 1989;12:1599–602.

[34] Swischuk LE. Irritable infant and left lower extremity pain. Pediatr Emerg Care 1997;13:147–8.

[35] Davison BL, Weinstein SL. Hip fractures in children: a long-term follow-up study. J Pediatr Orthop 1992;12:355–8.

[36] Miller WE. Fractures of the hip in children from birth to adolescence. Clin Orthop 1973;92:155–88.

[37] Togrul E, Bayram H, Gulsen M, et al. Fractures of the femoral neck in children: long-term follow-up in 62 hip fracture. Injury 2005;36:123–30.

[38] Wright JG, Wang EE, Owen JL, et al. Treatments for paediatric femoral fractures: a randomised trial. Lancet 2005;365:1153–8.

[39] Mass DP, Spiegel PG, Laros GS. Dislocation of the hip with traumatic separation of the capital femoral epiphysis: report of a case with successful outcome. Clin Orthop 1980;146:184–7.

[40] Raju KK, Tepler M, Dharapak C, et al. Transepiphyseal fracture of the hip in children. Orthop Rev 1984;13:65–77.

[41] Hoekstra HJ, Lichtendahl D. Pertrochanteric fractures in children and adolescents. J Pediatr Orthop 1983;3:587–91.

[42] Cheng JC, Tang N. Decompression and stable internal fixation of femoral neck fracture in children can affect the outcome. J Pediatr Orthop 1999;19:338–43.

[43] Maruenda JI, Barrios C, Gomar-Sancho F. Intracapsular hip pressure after femoral neck fracture. Clin Orthop 1997;340:172–80.

[44] Ng GP, Cole WG. Effect of early hip decompression on the frequency of avascular necrosis in children with fracture of the neck of the femur. Injury 1996;27:419–21.

[45] Song KS, Kim YS, Sohn SW, et al. Arthrotomy and open reduction of the displaced fracture of the femoral neck in children. J Pediatr Orthop B 2001;10B:205–10.

[46] Gerber C, Lehmann A, Ganz R. Femoral neck fractures in children: experience in 7 Swiss hospitals. Orthop Trans 1985;9:474.

[47] Ficat RP, Arlet J. Necroses of the femoral head. In: Ficat RP, Arlet J, Hungerford DS, editors. Ischemia and necroses of bone. Baltimore: Williams & Wilkins; 1980. p. 53–74.

[48] Marcus ND, Enneking WF, Massam RA. The silent hip in idiopathic aseptic necrosis: treatment by bone-grafting. J Bone Joint Surg Am 1973;55:1352–66.

[49] Steinberg ME, Hayken GD, Steinberg DR. A new method for evaluation and staging of avascular

[50] Plakseychuk AY, Shah M, Varitimidis SE, et al. Classification of osteonecrosis of the femoral head: reliability, reproducibility, and prognostic value. Clin Orthop 2001;386:34–41.

[51] Gardeniers JWM, Association Research Circulation Osseous Committee on Terminology and Staging. Report on the committee meeting at Santiago de Compostela. ARCO News 1993;5:79–82.

[52] Maeda S, Kita A, Fujii G, et al. Avascular necrosis associated with fractures of the femoral neck in children: histological evaluation of core biopsies of the femoral head. Injury 2003;34:283–6.

[53] Ovesen O, Arreskov J, Bellstrom T. Hip fractures in children: a long-term follow up of 17 cases. Orthopedics 1989;12:361–7.

[54] Lieberman JR. Core decompression for osteonecrosis of the hip. Clin Orthop 2004;418:29–33.

[55] Rijnen WH, Gardeniers JW, Buma P, et al. Treatment of femoral head osteonecrosis using bone impaction grafting. Clin Orthop 2003;417:74–83.

[56] Dean GS, Kime RC, Fitch RD, et al. Treatment of osteonecrosis in the hip of pediatric patients by free vascularized fibular graft. Clin Orthop 2001;386:106–13.

[57] Urbaniak JR, Coogan PE, Gunneson EB, et al. Treatment of osteonecrosis of the femoral head with free vascularized fibular grafting: a long-term follow-up study of one hundred and three hips. J Bone Joint Surg Am 1995;77:681–94.

[58] Adili A, Trousdale RT. Femoral head resurfacing for the treatment of osteonecrosis in the young patients. Clin Orthop 2003;417:93–101.

[59] Hungerford MW, Mont MA, Scott R, et al. Surface replacement hemiarthroplasty for the treatment of osteonecrosis of the femoral head. J Bone Joint Surg Am 1998;80:1656–64.

[60] Fulkerson JP. Arthrodesis for disabling hip pain in children and adolescents. Clin Orthop 1977;128:296–302.

[61] Taylor KF, McHale KA. Percutaneous pin fixation of a femoral neck fracture complicated by deep infection in a 12-year-old boy. Am J Orthop 2002;31:408–12.

[62] Forlin E, Guille JT, Kumar SJ, et al. Complications associated with fractures of the neck of the femur in children. J Pediatr Orthop 1992;12:503–9.

[63] Joseph B, Mulpuri K. Delayed separation of the capital femoral epiphysis after ipsilateral transcervical fractures of the femoral neck. J Orthop Trauma 2000;14:445–8.

Hip Arthroscopy in Children and Adolescents

Mininder S. Kocher, MD, MPH[a,b,]*, Ben Lee, BA[c]

[a]Division of Sports Medicine, Department of Orthopaedic Surgery, Children's Hospital, 300 Longwood Avenue, Boston, MA 02115, USA
[b]Harvard Medical School, Boston, MA, USA
[c]Department of Orthopaedic Surgery, Children's Hospital, 300 Longwood Avenue, Boston, MA 02115, USA

Described originally by Burman in 1931 [1], arthroscopy of the hip more recently has become an established procedure [2–6]. Arthroscopic surgery of the hip may offer potential advantages over traditional open arthrotomy and surgical dislocation in limited invasiveness and diminished morbidity. The most recognized indications for hip arthroscopy are for the management of labral tears [7–12] and loose bodies [8,13]. Hip arthroscopy has been described for a variety of other hip disorders, however, including osteoarthritis [8], osteonecrosis [8], osteochondral fracture [14], chondral injury [8], hip dysplasia [15], septic arthritis [16–18], inflammatory arthritis [8,19], synovial chondromatosis [20,21], foreign bodies [22], ligamentum tears [23–25], and complications after total joint arthroplasty [26–29].

Most of the experience in hip arthroscopy has been with hip disorders in adults. The indications and results of hip arthroscopy in children and adolescents have been less well characterized [14,19,30–35]. Pediatric hip conditions include Legg-Perthes disease, slipped capital femoral epiphysis, developmental dysplasia of the hip, septic arthritis, coxa vara, juvenile rheumatoid arthritis, and chondrolysis [36,37]. Gross described his early experience with hip arthroscopy in patients who had congenital dislocation of the hip, Legg-Perthes disease, slipped capital femoral epiphysis, and neuropathic subluxation [32]. Bowen and colleagues described arthroscopic chondroplasty of unstable osteochondral lesions of the femoral head as sequelae in patients after skeletal maturity who had Legg-Perthes disease as children [14,33]. Other indications in the pediatric population have included labral tears, loose bodies, chondral lesions, juvenile rheumatoid arthritis, and septic arthritis [19,30,31]. In a review of 24 hip arthroscopies performed in 21 patients aged 11 to 21 years, Schindler and colleagues concluded that hip arthroscopy was effective for synovial biopsy and loose body removal [34]. As a diagnostic procedure, however, the arthroscopy failed to correlate with the presumptive cause of symptoms in 11 hips (46%).

Technique

Hip arthroscopy can be performed in the supine or lateral decubitus position. Both positions allow for adequate visualization, and positioning typically is based on surgeon preference. Traction is used to distract the femoral head from the acetabulum, allowing for intra-articular access (Fig. 1). The authors perform hip arthroscopy in the supine position. The procedure is performed as an overnight observation procedure under general anesthesia with muscle relaxation. Fluoroscopy is used for establishment of portals. Specialized hip arthroscopy cannulae, motorized shavers, flexible tip electrocautery, baskets, and arthroscopic knives are used. Regular hip arthroscopy instrumentation can be used in adolescents and most older children. Specially sized instruments need to be developed to allow for hip arthroscopy in younger children. Anterolateral and posterolateral portals are

* Corresponding author. Division of Sports Medicine, Department of Orthopaedic Surgery, Children's Hospital, 300 Longwood Avenue, Boston, MA 02115.
E-mail address: mininder.kocher@childrens.harvard.edu (M.S. Kocher).

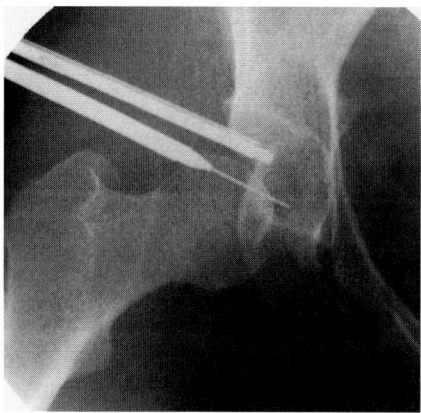

Fig. 1. Fluoroscopic image of hip arthroscopy with traction applied to allow insertion of arthroscope and instruments into the hip joint.

used routinely. The anterior portal is used infrequently. Thirty-degree and 70° arthroscopes routinely are used and switched between portals. Visualization is enhanced with the use of an arthroscopic fluid pump maintained at 60 mm Hg and addition of epinephrine to the arthroscopic fluid. Maneuverability within the joint is facilitated by performing small capsular releasing incisions with an arthroscopic knife.

Postoperative care depends on the specific procedure performed. Crutches typically are used for 14 days. Physical therapy is begun on the second postoperative day, emphasizing gentle range of motion, strength, pelvic tilts, and closed chain exercises as tolerated. Functional rehabilitation and return to unrestricted activities were progressed from 6 to 12 weeks, depending on the patient's symptoms and the diagnosis.

The authors recently reviewed our results of hip arthroscopy in children and adolescents [38,39]. From January 2001 to March 2004, 164 hip arthroscopies in 129 patients were performed by the first author in the Adolescent and Young Adult Hip Unit of Children's Hospital. Of these 164 procedures, 91 procedures were performed in 72 patients who were 18 years old and younger. Of these 91 procedures, 56 procedures in 44 patients had minimum 1-year follow-up. Two of these patients were lost to follow-up (follow-up rate, 95.5%). The study population thus included 54 hip arthroscopies in 42 patients.

Data collected included patient demographics, indications for surgery, complications, and outcome. Outcome was assessed preoperatively and postoperatively using the modified Harris Hip Score. The modified Harris Hip Score is a condition-specific outcome instrument that has been used widely after hip arthroscopy. The score assesses pain (44 points) and function (47 points). Function is divided into domains of limp (11 points), support (11 points), distance walked (11 points), stairs (4 points), socks/shoes (4 points), sitting (5 points), and public transportation (1 point). The modified Harris Hip Score was modified from the original by the elimination of the 9 points for range of motion and deformity because hip arthroscopy is indicated principally for pain and function. The modified Harris Hip Score thus is multiplied by 1.1 to give a total possible score of 100.

Mean patient age was 15.2 years (range, 5.9–18.9 years). Twenty-eight patients were female (67%) and 14 patients were male (33%). Minimum follow-up was 1 year, with mean 17.4-month follow-up (range, 12.0–26.2 months).

Chief complaints were pain in 48 hips and catching or locking in 6 hips. All patients reported diminished hip function. Fifteen patients had undergone 17 previous operations, including pelvic osteotomy (n = 11), femoral osteotomy (n = 5), and in situ pinning (n = 1). Indications for the 54 hip arthroscopies included isolated labral tears (n = 30), Perthes disease (n = 8), developmental dysplasia of the hip following prior periacetabular osteotomy (n = 8), inflammatory arthritis (n = 3), spondyloepiphyseal dysplasia (n = 2), avascular necrosis (n = 1), slipped capital femoral epiphysis (n = 1), and osteochondral fracture (n = 1). Specific procedures included debridement of labral tear (n = 41) (Figs. 2 and 3), chondroplasty of acetabulum or femoral head (n = 10) (Fig. 4), removal of loose bodies (n = 8) (Fig. 5), synovectomy (n = 3), and general debridement for degenerative changes (n = 2) (Fig. 6). Some hip arthroscopies included multiple specific components. Staged bilateral procedures were performed in nine patients. Revision procedures were performed in three patients who had recurrent labral tears. Concurrent procedures included iliotibial band release at the greater trochanter for snapping (n = 4) and proximal femoral blade plate removal (n = 1).

Overall there was significant improvement in modified Harris Hip Score (preoperative, 53.1; postoperative, 82.9; $P < 0.001$) (Table 1). For patients who had isolated labral tears (n = 30), there was significant improvement in modified Harris Hip Score (preoperative, 57.6; postoperative, 89.2; $P < 0.001$), and scores were improved in 26 of 30 procedures (Table 1). For patients who had Perthes disease (n = 8), there was significant improvement in modified Harris Hip Score (preoperative, 49.5; postoperative, 80.1; $P < 0.001$), and scores were improved in all eight procedures (Table 1). For patients who had labral tears with developmental dysplasia of the

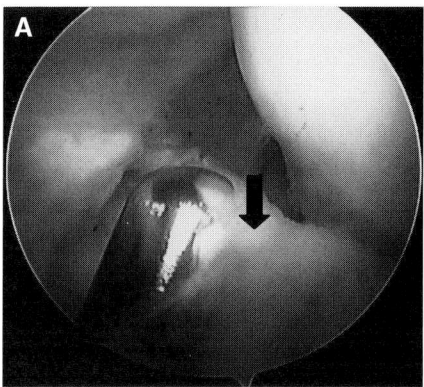 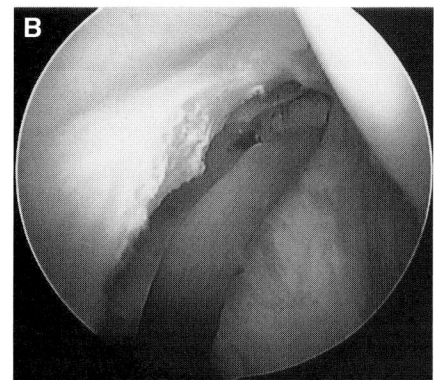

Fig. 2. Arthroscopic images of a longitudinal anterior labral tear (*arrow*). (*A*) Before debridement with arthroscopic shaver and (*B*) after debridement with radiofrequency ablation probe.

hip following prior periacetabular osteotomy (n = 8), there was significant improvement in modified Harris Hip Score (preoperative, 51.8; postoperative, 79.8; $P < 0.001$), and scores were improved in six of eight procedures (Table 1). For the two patients who had Outerbridge grade 4 degenerative changes (full-thickness chondral loss), scores were not improved. For patients who had inflammatory arthritis (n = 3), there was significant improvement in modified Harris Hip Score (preoperative, 54.8; postoperative, 81.3; $P < 0.001$), and scores were improved in all three procedures (Table 1). Preoperative and postoperative modified Harris Hip Scores for patients who had spondyloepiphyseal dysplasia (n = 2), avascular necrosis (n = 1), slipped femoral capital epiphysis (n = 1), and osteochondral fracture (n = 1) are shown in Table 1.

Complications included transient pudendal nerve palsy (n = 3), instrument breakage (n = 1), and recurrent labral tear (n = 3). All three patients who had pudendal nerve palsies had paresthesia in the groin and scrotal/labial region that resolved spontaneously by 3 months postoperatively. The case of instrument breakage involved shearing off of a flexible guide wire by a cannulated obturator on insertion. The broken guide wire was retrieved arthroscopically. Two patients who had isolated labral tears and one patient who had developmental dysplasia of the hip following prior periacetabular osteotomy who had undergone arthroscopic debridement had recurrent labral tears (recurrent labral tear rate, 3 of 41 [7.3%]). All three patients had demonstrated improvement after their initial arthroscopic debridement, with recurrent symptoms developing 3 to 21 months after their index procedure. All three patients improved after repeat arthroscopy and labral tear debridement.

In reviewing our results of hip arthroscopy in children and adolescents for various diagnoses, hip arthroscopy thus was a safe procedure with few com-

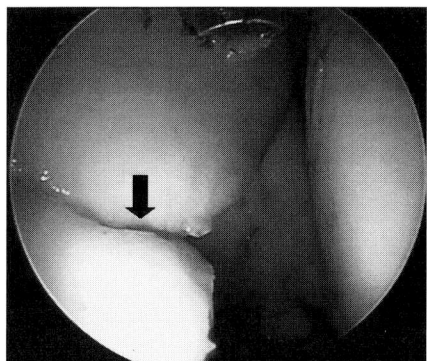

Fig. 3. Arthroscopic image of a radial anterior labral tear (*arrow*).

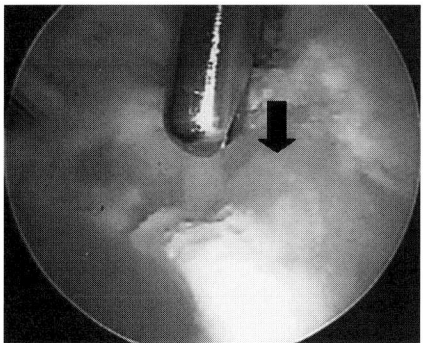

Fig. 4. Chondroplasty of an anterior acetabular chondral flap (*arrow*).

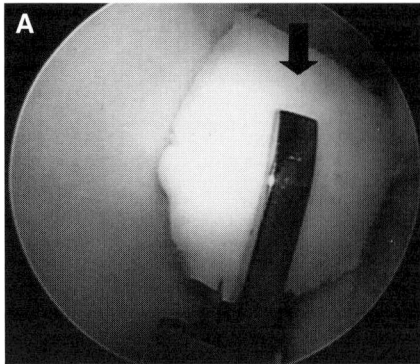 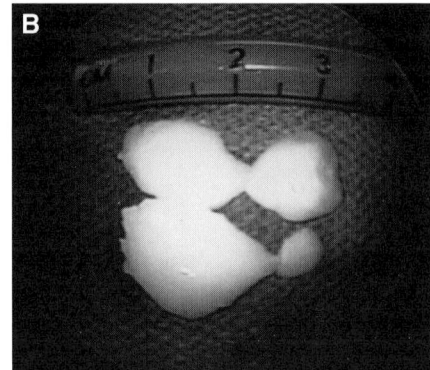

Fig. 5. Loose bodies associated with spondyloepiphyseal dysplasia. (*A*) Arthroscopic image of intra-articular loose body (*arrow*) held by grasper. (*B*) Multiple loose bodies after removal.

plications and appeared efficacious in the short term for certain indications.

Specific indications

Labral tears

The acetabular labrum is a thin fibrocartilaginous rim surrounding the acetabulum and acts to deepen the acetabulum and enhance articular congruency. Conflicting evidence exists regarding the biomechanical role of the acetabular labrum. Although a study by Konrath and colleagues [40] demonstrated that the labrum does not play a fundamental role in load transmission through the hip, a more recent study by Peterson and colleagues [41] found that excision or removal of the labrum following trauma could adversely affect joint stability and load distribution.

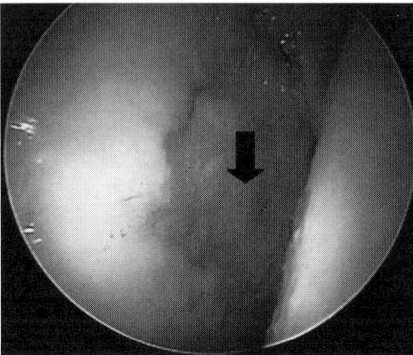

Fig. 6. Full thickness cartilage loss (*arrow*) of the anterosuperior acetabulum in a patient who had hip dysplasia after prior periacetabular osteotomy.

During the same study, Petersen also assessed the vascularity of the labrum, demonstrating that only the peripheral third of the labrum receives a vascular supply from the adjacent joint capsule, leaving the internal two thirds avascular [41]. Consequently tears occurring at watershed zones can cause destabilization of the adjacent acetabular cartilage, and if left untreated have been demonstrated with the use of MRA to progress eventually to osteoarthritis [42–44].

Acetabular labrum tears are common among athletes and typically occur anteriorly. In a review on the topic, Hickman and Peters attribute more than 60% of all labral tears to a traumatic event or to acetabular dysplasias, such as developmental dysplasia, Legg-Calve-Perthes disease, neuropathic subluxation of the hip, or previous episodes of septic arthritis [44]. The mechanism of injury generally involves repetitive twisting or pivoting movements resulting in hyperextension, hyperflexion, or extremes of abduction [45]. Presentation classically involves acute onset unilateral hip pain or alternatively insidious hip pain that escalates over time. Associated mechanical symptoms are present in almost all cases [16,45]. A study conducted by Narvani and colleagues demonstrated that a clicking sensation of the hip was 100% sensitive and 85% specific for predicting labral tears [46]. Furthermore, the internal rotation-flexion-axial compression test was 75% sensitive and 43% specific [40]. The Thomas test was neither sensitive nor specific [46].

Accurate diagnosis and treatment of acetabular labral tears is important not only to provide relief from pain but also in the prevention of subsequent osteoarthritis [44]. With the advent of MR arthrography (Fig. 7) and the increasing popularity of hip arthroscopy (see Figs. 2 and 3), this diagnostic and therapeutic challenge has been reduced significantly [44].

Table 1
Modified Harris Hip Score results by diagnosis

Diagnosis	n	Preoperative	Postoperative	p Value
Overall	54	53.1 (7.3)	82.9 (8.1)	<0.001
Isolated labral tear	30	57.6 (7.2)	89.2 (8.5)	<0.001
Perthes disease	8	49.5 (7.7)	80.1 (7.9)	<0.001
Developmental dysplasia of the hip (after prior periacetabular osteotomy)	8	51.8 (8.1)	79.8 (8.9)	<0.001
Inflammatory arthritis	3	54.8 (7.0)	81.3 (8.2)	<0.001
Spondyloepiphyseal dysplasia	2	47.5	82.5	—
Avascular necrosis	1	55	55	—
Slipped capital femoral epiphysis	1	62	85	—
Osteochondral fracture	1	29	96	—

Values represent mean (standard deviation).

First-line management typically involves nonoperative interventions, such as the use of nonsteroidal anti-inflammatory drugs and partial weightbearing; however, surgical intervention ultimately is required in most cases because of continued pain and mechanical symptoms [44].

Although the success of open arthrotomy and labral debridement is well documented in the literature, the use of arthroscopic labral debridement is increasing in popularity, because it provides a safe and minimally invasive treatment alternative to open arthrotomy when conservative management fails [44]. Three independent studies by Farjo and colleagues [47], Hase and colleagues [48], and Lage and colleagues [49] have demonstrated that careful debridement of the torn labrum back to a stable base, while preserving the capsular labral tissue, effectively relieves pain and eliminates mechanical symptoms in those patients who have no associated degenerative hip changes. Unfortunately in patients in whom dysplastic or degenerative changes of the hip have been documented preoperatively, there was no improvement in symptoms or hip function observed [47–49]. This is significant, because in a study conducted by Wenger and colleagues of 31 patients who had acetabular labral tears, 87% (27 of 31) had at least one structural hip abnormality on conventional radiograph, and 35% had more than one abnormality [50]. Not only does pre-existing degenerative or dysplastic hip disease predispose to acetabular labral tears, but it thus also has a major impact on treatment outcome and long-term prognosis [50].

Developmental dysplasia of the hip

Intra-articular pathology often is associated with developmental dysplasia of the hip [36,37,51]. Hip dysplasia may present in adolescence or young adulthood as hip pain from a degenerative labral tear or chondral lesion. Anterior labral tears also may occur as a result of anterior impingement from a post-slipped capital femoral epiphysis deformity or pistol-grip deformity [35,52]. Although favorable results have been reported from the arthroscopic management of intra-articular pathology in dysplastic hips [9], the authors' preferred approach is to address the underlying dysplasia with periacetabular osteotomy with or without proximal femoral osteotomy [36,37]. After periacetabular osteotomy, some patients may present with increasing hip pain and mechanical symptoms caused by a degenerative labral tear. In our series, the authors found improvement in symptoms with arthroscopic debridement in six of eight patients. The two patients who had full-thickness degenerative joint disease did not improve after arthroscopic debridement, however, questioning its efficacy in patients who have advanced degenerative joint disease.

Loose bodies

Loose bodies of the hip may occur from traumatic injury (Fig. 8) or as a sequela of hip disorders, such as

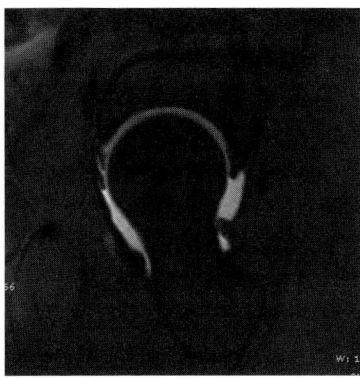

Fig. 7. MR arthrogram demonstrating an anterior labral tear.

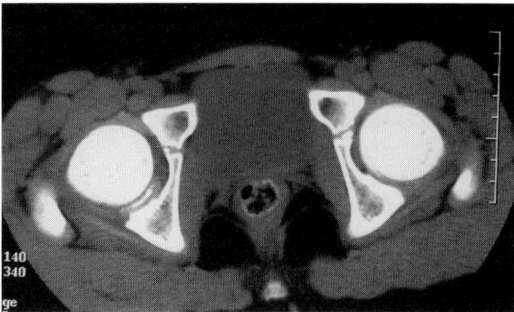

Fig. 8. CT scan demonstrating intra-articular loose body in the right hip after traumatic posterior hip dislocation.

Legg-Perthes disease, spondyloepiphyseal dysplasia, chondrocalcinosis, or avascular necrosis. In patients who have Legg-Perthes disease, an unstable osteochondral fragment in the central portion of the femoral head may persist after the healing phase, particularly in patients who have a flattened, aspherical head. Patients may present with pain and mechanical symptoms, such as catching or locking. The loose osteochondral lesions may be visible on radiographs, CT scan, or MRI. Arthroscopic excision has yielded excellent results with minimal morbidity [8,13]. In the authors' series, loose bodies were associated with Legg-Perthes disease, spondyloepiphyseal dysplasia, and traumatic osteochondral fracture, and excision typically resulted in resolution of pain and mechanical symptoms during this period of follow-up. The longer-term prognosis in patients who have Legg-Perthes disease remains guarded, however, if there is substantial asphericity of the femoral head [36,37].

Inflammatory arthritis/septic arthritis

Arthroscopic synovectomy of the hip in cases of inflammatory arthritis has been suggested to improve pain and function [19]. In this series, three patients who had inflammatory arthritis underwent arthroscopic synovectomy for hip pain and dysfunction that was recalcitrant to medical therapy, and all three patients demonstrated improvement.

Arthroscopic irrigation and debridement of septic arthritis of the hip in children has been reported [16–18]. The authors' preference is for open arthrotomy through a limited anterior approach to the hip, because this allows for capsulectomy, drilling of the femoral neck to rule out associated osteomyelitis, thorough debridement of infected tissue, and placement of a drain.

Other indications

Femoroacetabular impingement is a condition that is being further developed and understood. CAM-type and pincer-type impingement can result in degenerative joint disease. Arthroscopic management of femoroacetabular impingement has recently received attention.

Arthroscopy potentially may be used as an adjunct during closed reduction for hip dysplasia in infants. Arthroscopy may allow for the visualization of impediments to reduction, transection of the transverse acetabular ligament, and assessment of reduction.

Complications

Reported complications of hip arthroscopy include iatrogenic injury to the articular surfaces, pudendal nerve palsy, lateral femoral cutaneous nerve injury, femoral nerve injury, sciatic nerve injury, femoral artery injury, intrapelvic fluid extravasation, skin pressure ulcers from traction, heterotopic ossification, instrument breakage, infection, and deep venous thrombosis [2–6,53,54]. In the authors' series, there were minimal complications. The three cases of pudendal nerve paresthesias resolved spontaneously within 3 months of surgery. One broken guide wire was retrieved arthroscopically. Repeat surgery for recurrent labral tears was necessary in 7% (3 of 41) of index labral tear procedures.

Summary

Hip arthroscopy offers potential advantages over traditional open arthrotomy and surgical dislocation in limited invasiveness and diminished morbidity. Most of the experience in hip arthroscopy has been with hip disorders in adults. The indications and results of hip arthroscopy in children and adolescents have been less well characterized. The pediatric hip has unique conditions, including Legg-Perthes disease, slipped capital femoral epiphysis, developmental dysplasia of the hip, septic arthritis, coxa vara, juvenile rheumatoid arthritis, and chondrolysis. Hip arthroscopy in children and adolescents may be efficacious for certain indications, including isolated labral tears, loose bodies, and chondral flaps associated with Legg-Perthes diseases or spondyloepiphyseal dysplasia, labral tears associated with hip dysplasia after prior periacetabular osteotomy, and inflammatory arthritis. Further development of hip arthroscopy in children and adolescents is necessary to refine indications, evaluate longer-term results, and develop pediatric-specific instrumentation.

References

[1] Burman MS. Arthroscopy or the direct visualization of joints. J Bone Joint Surg Am 1931;13:669–95.

[2] Byrd JWT. Indications and contraindications. In: Byrd JWT, editor. Operative hip arthroscopy. New York: Thieme; 1998. p. 7–24.

[3] Frich LH, Lauritzen J, Juhl M. Arthroscopy in diagnosis and treatment of hip disorders. Orthopedics 1989; 12:389–92.

[4] Ide T, Akamatsu N, Nakajima I. Arthroscopic surgery of the hip joint. Arthroscopy 1991;7:204–11.

[5] McCarthy JC, Day B, Busconi B. Hip arthroscopy: applications and techniques. J Am Acad Orthop Surg 1995;3:115–22.

[6] Parisien S. Arthroscopy of the hip. Present status. J Dis Orthop 1985;45:127–32.

[7] Byrd JWT. Labral lesions: an elusive source of hip pain: case reports and review of the literature. Arthroscopy 1996;12:603–12.

[8] Byrd JWT, Jones KS. Prospective analysis of hip arthroscopy with 2-year follow-up. Arthroscopy 2000; 16:578–87.

[9] Byrd JWT, Jones KS. Hip arthroscopy in the presence of dysplasia. Arthroscopy 2003;19:1055–60.

[10] Dorell JH, Catterall A. The torn acetabular labrum. J Bone Joint Surg [Br] 1986;68:400–3.

[11] Suzuki S, Awaya G, Okada Y, et al. Arthroscopic diagnosis of ruptured acetabular labrum. Acta Orthop Scand 1986;57:513–5.

[12] Villar RN. Arthroscopic debridement of the hip. J Bone Joint Surg [Br] 1991;73:170–1.

[13] Byrd JWT. Hip arthroscopy for post-traumatic loose fragments in the young active adult: three case reports. Clin Sports Med 1996;6:129–34.

[14] Bowen JR, Kumar VP, Joyce III JJ, et al. Osteochondritis dissecans following Perthes' disease. Arthroscopic operative treatment. Clin Orthop 1986;209:49–56.

[15] Noguchi Y, Miura H, Takasugi S, et al. Cartilage and labrum degeneration in the dysplastic hip generally originates in the anterosuperior weight bearing area: an arthroscopic observation. Arthroscopy 1999;15: 496–506.

[16] Blitzer CM. Arthroscopic management of septic arthritis of the hip. Arthroscopy 1993;9:414–6.

[17] Bould M, Edwards D, Villar RN. Arthroscopic diagnosis and treatment of septic arthritis of the hip joint. Arthroscopy 1993;9:707–8.

[18] Chung WK, Slater GL, Bates EH. Treatment of septic arthritis of the hip by arthroscopic lavage. J Pediatr Orthop 1993;13:444–6.

[19] Holgersson S, Brattstr MH, Mogensen B, et al. Arthroscopy of the hip in juvenile chronic arthritis. J Pediatr Orthop 1981;1:273–8.

[20] Okada Y, Awaya G, Ikeda T, et al. Arthroscopic surgery for synovial chondromatosis of the hip. J Bone Joint Surg [Br] 1989;71:198–9.

[21] Witwity T, Uhlmann RD, Fischer J. Arthroscopic management of chondromatosis of the hip joint. Arthroscopy 1988;4:55–6.

[22] Goldman A, Minkoff J, Price A, et al. A posterior arthroscopic approach to bullet extraction from the hip. J Trauma 1987;27:1294–300.

[23] Delcamp DD, Klaaren HE, Pompe van Meerdervoort HF. Traumatic avulsion of the ligamentum teres without dislocation of the hip. J Bone Joint Surg [Am] 1988;70:933–5.

[24] Gray AJR, Villar RN. The ligamentum teres of the hip: an arthroscopic classification of its pathology. Arthroscopy 1997;13:575–8.

[25] Kashiwagi N, Suzuki S, Seto Y. Arthroscopic treatment for traumatic hip dislocation with avulsion fracture of the ligamentum teres. Arthroscopy 2001;17:67–9.

[26] Mah ET, Bradley CM. Arthroscopic removal of acrylic cement from unreduced hip prosthesis. Aust N Z J Surg 1992;62:508–10.

[27] Nordt W, Giangarra CE, Levy I, et al. Arthroscopic removal of entrapped debris following dislocation of a total hip arthroplasty. Arthroscopy 1987;3:196–8.

[28] Shifrin LZ, Reis ND. Arthroscopy of a dislocated hip replacement: a case report. Clin Orthop 1978;6:213–4.

[29] Vakili F, Salvati EA, Warren RF. Entrapped foreign body within the acetabular cup in total hip replacement. Clin Orthop 1980;150:159–62.

[30] Berend KR, Vail TP. Hip arthroscopy in the adolescent and pediatric athlete. Clin Sports Med 2001;20:763–8.

[31] DeAngelis NA, Busconi BD. Hip arthroscopy in the pediatric population. Clin Orthop 2003;406:60–3.

[32] Gross RH. Arthroscopy in hip disorders in children. Orthop Rev 1977;6:43–9.

[33] Lechevallier J, Bowen JR. Arthroscopic treatment of the late sequelae of Legg-Calve-Perthes disease. J Bone Joint Surg [Br] 1993;75(Suppl 2):160–5.

[34] Schindler A, Lechevallier JJ, Rao NS, et al. Diagnostic and therapeutic arthroscopy of the hip in children and adolescents: evaluation of results. J Pediatr Orthop 1995;15:317–21.

[35] Snow SW, Keret D, Scarangella S, et al. Anterior impingement of the femoral head: a late phenomenon of Legg-Calvé-Perthes' disease. J Pediatr Orthop 1993; 13:286–9.

[36] Millis MB, Kocher MS. Hip, pelvis, femur: pediatric aspects. In: Koval KJ, editor. Orthopaedic knowledge update 7. Chicago: American Academy of Orthopaedic Surgeons; 2002. p. 387–94.

[37] Millis MB, Kocher MS. Hip and pelvic injuries in the young athlete (section B). 2nd edition. In: DeLee J, Drez D, Miller MD, editors. DeLee & Drez's orthopaedic sports medicine: principles and practice, Vol. 2. Philadelphia: Saunders; 2003. p. 1463–79.

[38] Kocher MS, Kim YJ, Millis MB, et al. Hip arthroscopy in children and adolescents. J Pediatr Orthop 2005; 25:680–6.

[39] Millis MB, Kocher MS. Hip and pelvic injuries in the young athlete. In: Miller M, editor. Pediatric and adolescent sports medicine. 2nd edition. Philadelphia: WB Saunders Co.; 2002. p. 175–84.

[40] Konrath GA, Amel AJ, Olson SA, et al. The role of the acetabular labrum and the transverse acetabular ligament in load transmission in the hip. J Bone Joint Surg [Am] 1998;80:1781.

[41] Petersen W, Petersen F, Tillmann B. Structure and vascularization of the acetabular labrum with regards to the pathogenesis and healing of labral tears. Arch Orthop Trauma Surg 2003;123(6):283–8.

[42] McCarthy J, Noble P, Aluisio FV, et al. Anatomy, pathologic features and treatment of acetabular labrum tears. Clin Orthop 2003;406:38–47.

[43] McCarthy JC, Noble PC, Schuck MR, et al. The Watershed labral lesion: its relationship to early arthritis of the hip. J Arthroplasty 2001;16(8, suppl 1):81–7.

[44] Hickman JM, Peters CL. Hip pain in the young adult: diagnosis and treatment of disorders of the acetabular labrum and acetabular dysplasia. Am J Orthop 2001; 30(6):459–67.

[45] Mason JB. Acetabular labral tears in the athlete. Clin Sports Med 2001;20(4):779–90.

[46] Narvani AA, Tsiridis E, Kendall S, et al. A preliminary report on prevalence of acetabular labrum tears in sports patients with groin pain. Knee Surg Sports Traumatol Arthrosc 2003;11(6):403–8.

[47] Farjo LA, Glick JM, Sampson TG. Hip arthroscopy for acetabular labral tears. Arthroscopy 1999;1:132–7.

[48] Hase T, Ueo T. Acetabular labral tear: arthroscopic diagnosis and treatment. Arthroscopy 1999;15:138–41.

[49] Lage LA, Patel JV, Villar RN. The acetabular labral tear: an arthroscopic classification. Arthroscopy 1999; 15:269–72.

[50] Wenger DE, Kendell KR, Miner MR, et al. Acetabular labral tears rarely occur in the absence of bony abnormalities. Clin Orthop 2004;426:145–50.

[51] Cooperman DR, Wallensten R, Stulberg SD. Acetabular dysplasia in the adult. Clin Orthop 1983;175: 79–85.

[52] Klaue K, Durnin CW, Ganz R. The acetabular rim syndrome. J Bone Joint Surg [Br] 1991;73B:423–9.

[53] Byrd JWT. Complications associated with hip arthroscopy. In: Byrd JWT, editor. Operative hip arthroscopy. New York: Thieme; 1998. p. 171–6.

[54] Funke EL, Munzinger U. Complications in hip arthroscopy. Arthroscopy 1996;12:156–9.

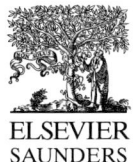

Index

Note: Page numbers of article titles are in **boldface** type.

A

Acetabular procedure
  for DDH in children, 151–152

Adolescent(s)
  hip arthroscopy in, **233–240**. See also *Hip arthroscopy, in children and adolescents.*

Age
  as factor in DDH treatment in children, 150

Arthritis
  inflammatory
    hip arthroscopy for, 238
  septic. See *Septic arthritis.*

Arthroplasty
  greater trochanteric
    for septic arthritis of hip, 176

Avascular necrosis
  after surgical treatment for DDH in children, 155–156
  unstable SCFE and, 214–216

B

Bone graft epiphysiodesis
  in unstable SCFE management, 214

C

Cell signaling
  in intrauterine joint development, 122–123

Cerebral palsy
  hip dysplasia in, **185–196**
    evaluation of
      physical examination in, 186
      radiologic, 186–187
    natural history of, 187–189
    pathophysiology of, 185–186

  treatment of
    nonoperative, 189
    surgical, 189–193
      osseous reconstruction in, 191–193

Charcot-Marie-Tooth disease
  clinical presentation of, 203–204
  described, 203
  genetic defects in, 203
  hip dysplasia in, **203–209**
    described, 204–205
    evaluation of, 205–206
    treatment of, 206–208
  type 1, 203
  type 2, 203

Children
  DDH in
    treatment of, **149–160**. See also *Developmental dysplasia of hip (DDH), in children, treatment of.*
  hip arthroscopy in, **233–240**. See also *Hip arthroscopy, in children and adolescents.*
  hip fractures in, **223–232**. See also *Hip(s), fractures of, in children.*
  hip(s) of. See *Hip(s), of children.*
  SCFE in
    fixation for, 219
    unilateral
      prophylactic fixation of contralateral hip for, 218–219
  spinal cord injuries in
    hip disorders with, **197–202**. See also *Hip disorders, in children with spinal cord injuries.*
    prevalence of, 197
    treatment of
      principles of, 197

Contracture(s)
  joint
    in children with spinal cord injuries, 201

Cox vara
  hip fractures in children and, 229

D

DDH. See *Developmental dysplasia of hip (DDH)*.

Developmental dysplasia of hip (DDH), 128–130, **141–147**
- diagnosis of
  - ultrasound in, 141–144
    - advantages of, 142
    - in hip joint screening, 142–144
    - person performing, 144
- in children
  - treatment of, **149–160**
    - acetabular procedure in, 151–152
    - age limit for, 150
    - avascular necrosis after, 155–156
    - complications of, 155–158
    - femoral shortening in, 150–151, 153
    - goals in, 149
    - indication for, 149–150
    - open reduction in, 150, 152
    - options for, 150–152
    - osteoarthritis after, 157–158
    - redislocation after, 156
    - residual dysplasia after, 156–157
    - results of, 655
    - stiffness after, 156
  - treatment of
    - arthroscopy in, 237
    - ultrasound in, 144–146

Dysplasia(s)
- developmental
  - of hip, **141–147**. See also *Developmental dysplasia of hip (DDH)*.
- hip
  - in cerebral palsy, **185–196**. See also *Cerebral palsy, hip dysplasia in*.
  - in Charcot-Marie-Tooth disease, **203–209**. See also *Charcot-Marie-Tooth disease, hip dysplasia in*.
- residual
  - after surgical treatment for DDH in children, 156–157

E

Epiphysiodesis
- bone graft
  - in unstable SCFE management, 214

F

Femoral shortening
- for DDH in children, 150–151, 153

Fracture(s)
- hip
  - in children, **223–232**. See also *Hip(s), fractures of, in children*.
- pathologic
  - in children with spinal cord injuries, 201–202

G

Ganz osteotomy
- for late hip dysplasia, **161–171**
  - patient outcomes after, 167–170
  - procedure, 164–167

Genetic defects
- in Charcot-Marie-Tooth disease, 203

Greater trochanteric arthroplasty
- for septic arthritis of hip, 176

H

Harcke's method
- in ultrasound examination of DDH, 141

Hereditary motor and sensory neuropathy, **203–209**. See also *Charcot-Marie-Tooth disease*.

Heterotopic ossification
- in children with spinal cord injuries, 201

Hip(s)
- anatomy of
  - in children, 223
- developmental dysplasia of, **141–147**. See also *Developmental dysplasia of hip (DDH)*.
- dislocation of
  - abnormalities associated with, 149
- disorders of. See *Hip disorders*.
- fractures of
  - in children, **223–232**
    - classification of, 224–226
    - complications of, 228–230
    - diagnosis of, 224
    - mechanism of injury, 223–224
    - treatment of, 226–228
    - type I, 224–225
    - type II, 225–226
    - type III, 226
    - type IV, 226
- of children
  - anatomy of, 223
  - arterial supply to
    - development of, 125
  - growth and development of, **119–132**
    - abnormal, 128–131
      - DDH, 128–130
      - Legg-Calvé-Perthes disease, 130–131

acetabular, 123–124
femoral anteversion in, 121–122
intrauterine joint development
cell signaling in, 122–123
limb position in, 121–122
neck-shaft angle in, 121–122
postnatal, 123–124
prenatal cellular development, 119–121
proximal femoral development, 124–128
pain related to. See *Hip pain, in children.*
pain related to. See *Hip pain.*
septic arthritis of
operative reconstruction for, **173–183.**
See also *Septic arthritis, of hip, operative reconstruction for.*
subluxation/dislocation of
in children with spinal cord injuries, 197–201
ultrasound of
in DDH diagnosis
advantages of, 142

Hip arthroscopy
in children and adolescents, **233–240**
complications of, 238
indications for, 235–238
DDH, 237
inflammatory arthritis/septic arthritis, 238
labral tears, 235–237
loose bodies, 237–238
technique of, 233–235

Hip disorders
in children and adolescents
types of, 233
in children with spinal cord injuries, **197–197**
heterotopic ossification, 201
hip subluxation/dislocation, 197–201
joint contractures, 201
pathologic fractures, 201–202

Hip dysplasia
described, 161–162
in cerebral palsy, **185–196.** See also *Cerebral palsy, hip dysplasia in.*
in Charcot-Marie-Tooth disease, **203–209.**
See also *Charcot-Marie-Tooth disease, hip dysplasia in.*
late
evaluation of, 162–164
Ganz osteotomy for, **161–171**
patient outcomes after, 167–170
procedure, 164–167

Hip joints
DDH and
screening of
ultrasound in, 142–144

Hip pain
in children
causes of, 135–138
infectious, 136–138
inflammatory, 136–138
mechanical, 135–136
traumatic, 135–136
vascular, 138
evaluation of, **133–140**
imaging in, 135
laboratory studies in, 134–135
patient history in, 133–134
physical examination in, 134
neoplastic conditions and, 138–139

I

Inflammatory arthritis
hip arthroscopy for, 238

Intrauterine joint
development of
cell signaling in, 122–123

J

Joint(s)
hip
DDH and
screening of
ultrasound in, 142–144
intrauterine
development of
cell signaling in, 122–123

Joint contractures
in children with spinal cord injuries, 201

L

Labral tears
hip arthroscopy for, 235–237

Legg-Calvé-Perthes disease, 130–131

Loose bodies
hip arthroscopy for, 237–238

N

Neoplastic conditions
hip pain in children due to, 138–139

Nonunion
hip fractures in children and, 229–230

O

Open reduction
    for DDH in children, 150, 152

Osseous reconstruction
    for hip dysplasia in cerebral palsy, 191–193

Osteoarthritis
    after surgical treatment for DDH in children, 157–158

Osteonecrosis
    hip fractures in children and, 228–229

Osteotomy(ies)
    for SCFE, 216–218
    Ganz
        for late hip dysplasia, **161–171**
            patient outcomes after, 167–170
            procedure, 164–167
    pelvic support
        for septic arthritis of hip, 176–181

P

Pain
    hip
        in children. See also *Hip pain, in children.*

Palsy(ies)
    cerebral
        hip dysplasia in, **185–196.** See also *Cerebral palsy, hip dysplasia in.*

Pelvic support osteotomy
    for septic arthritis of hip, 176–181

Premature physeal closure
    hip fractures in children and, 229

R

Redislocation
    after surgical treatment for DDH in children, 156

S

SCFE. See *Slipped capital femoral epiphysis (SCFE).*

Septic arthritis
    of hip
        arthroscopy for, 238
        late sequelae of
            radiographic classifications of, 173–175
                type I, 173–174
                type II, 174–175
                type III, 175
                type IV, 175
        operative reconstruction for, **173–183**
            algorithmic treatment strategy for, 175–176
            greater trochanteric arthroplasty in, 176
            pelvic support osteotomy in, 176–181

Slipped capital femoral epiphysis (SCFE)
    classification of, 211
    controversies in, **211–221**
    hip pain in children due to, 135–136
    in children
        fixation in, 219
    stable *vs.* unstable, 211
    treatment of
        osteotomy in, 216–218
    unilateral
        in children
            prophylactic fixation of contralateral hip for, 218–219
    unstable
        avascular necrosis due to, 214–216
        complications of, 214–216
        treatment of, 211–216
            bone graft epiphysiodesis in, 214
            in situ fixation in, 213
            internal fixation in, 213
            mini-arthrotomy for joint depression in, 213
            two-screw fixation in, 213
        vs. stable, 211

Spinal cord injuries
    in children
        hip disorders and, **197–197.** See also *Hip disorders, in children with spinal cord injuries.*
        prevalence of, 197
        treatment of
            principles of, 197

Stiffness
    after surgical treatment for DDH in children, 156

U

Ultrasound
    in DDH diagnosis, 141–144. See also *Developmental dysplasia of hip (DDH), diagnosis of, ultrasound in.*
    in DDH management, 144–146

Changing Your Address?

Make sure your subscription changes too! When you notify us of your new address, you can help make our job easier by including an exact copy of your Clinics label number with your old address (see illustration below.) This number identifies you to our computer system and will speed the processing of your address change. Please be sure this label number accompanies your old address and your corrected address—you can send an old Clinics label with your number on it or just copy it exactly and send it to the address listed below.

We appreciate your help in our attempt to give you continuous coverage. Thank you.

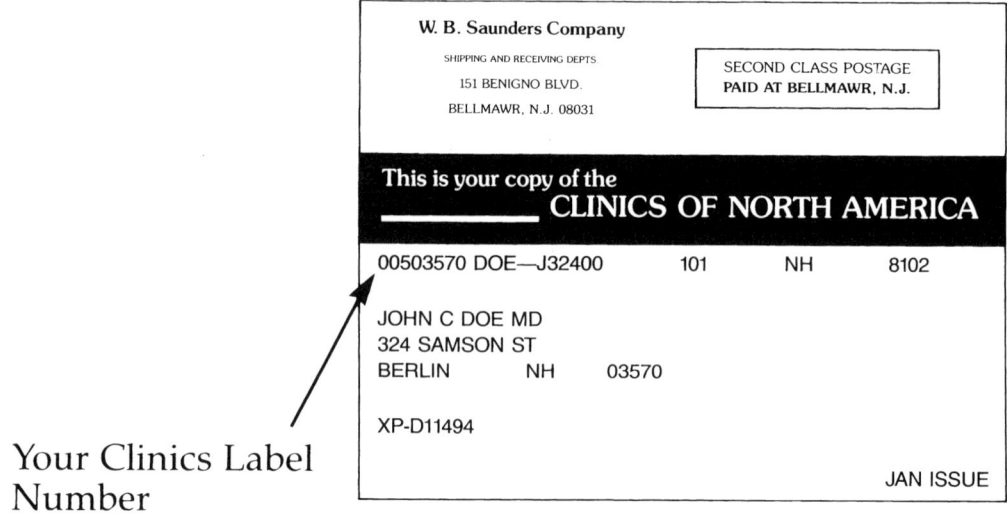

Your Clinics Label Number
Copy it exactly or send your label along with your address to:
W.B. Saunders Company, Customer Service
Orlando, FL 32887-4800
Call Toll Free 1-800-654-2452

Please allow four to six weeks for delivery of new subscriptions and for processing address changes.